616.86 Schr
Schneider,
Cybersex exposed
c2001

13   3/06
16 4/07

MB

Cybersex Exposed

Cybersex Exposed

Simple Fantasy or Obsession?

Jennifer Schneider, M.D., Ph.D.
Robert Weiss, M.S.W., C.A.S.

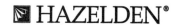 HAZELDEN®

INFORMATION & EDUCATIONAL SERVICES

Hazelden
Center City, Minnesota 55012-0176

1-800-328-0094
1-651-213-4590 (Fax)
www.hazelden.org

© 2001 by Jennifer Schneider and Robert Weiss
All rights reserved. Published 2001
Printed in the United States of America
No portion of this publication may be reproduced in any manner
without the written permission of the publisher

Library of Congress Cataloging-in-Publication Data
Schneider, Jennifer P.
   Cybersex exposed : simple fantasy or obsession? / Jennifer Schneider,
     Robert Weiss.   p. cm.
Includes bibliographical references and index.
ISBN 1-56838-619-2
   1. Sex addiction. 2. Computer sex. I. Weiss, Robert, 1961– II. Title.

RC560.S43 S358 2001
616.86—dc21
                                                                         00-054209

The Women's Sexual Addiction Screening Test (W-SAST) on pages 194–195 is copy-righted © 1999 by SexHelp.com. It is reprinted with the permission of SexHelp.com.

Author's note
Every story in this book is true; however, each has been edited for clarity. Names, loca-tions, and other identifying information have been changed to protect confidentiality.

Editor's note
The Twelve Steps of Sexual Compulsives Anonymous (SCA), as adapted by SCA with permission of Alcoholics Anonymous World Services, Inc. (AAWS), are reprinted with permission of SCA and AAWS. The Twelve Steps of Alcoholics Anonymous are reprinted with the permission of AAWS. AAWS's permission to reprint the foregoing material does not mean that AAWS has reviewed or approved the contents of this pub-lication, or that AAWS necessarily agrees with the views expressed herein. Alcoholics Anonymous is a program of recovery from alcoholism *only*—use or permissible adapta-tion of AA's Twelve Steps in connection with programs and activities which are pat-terned after AA, but which address other problems, or in any other non-AA context, does not imply otherwise. SCA and AA are not affiliated in any way.

05 04 03 02 01   6 5 4 3 2 1

Cover design by Stephen Clement
Interior design by Elizabeth Cleveland
Typesetting by Stanton Publication Services, Inc.

*To those struggling with their secrets—hidden from those
they might love—we dedicate this book in the hope
that they will find their way home.*

Contents

Preface

This book arose from the many exchanges both of us have had with people troubled by their online sexual behavior. As writers and facilitators of sex addiction and co-addiction treatment, over the years we have seen how sex addicts have experimented with the various popular trends in sexuality only to integrate these new behaviors into their destructive repertoire. From newspaper personals to phone sex and now the Internet, we have observed the passing trends, noting that even as the methods of delivery of sex have changed, addictive behavior patterns remain constant. The reason online sex has caught our attention has to do with how pervasive and intensely addictive this type of sexual connection has proved to be. Just as recreational use of certain drugs, such as nicotine and cocaine, tends to escalate to addictive use more rapidly than does experimentation with other drugs, so has Internet sex and its online connections proven to be an almost instant source of addiction for some people.

Because attitudes on sexuality are often considered to be a reflection of one's attitudes on morality, we want to state clearly our position on sexual behavior, sexual orientation, and attitudes toward sex. We, the authors, entirely support each person in his or her right to engage in whatever type of sexual activity and experience that provides both them and their partners pleasure, satisfaction, and fulfillment. We do not believe that we or anyone else has the right to judge or discriminate against a person's sexual decisions, provided that those choices do not violate the intrinsic rights and safety of others. We also respect and believe in the rights of children not to be exposed to sexually oriented material or exploitation. Our work is not focused on what is morally correct for people or the culture at large. We are not "sex-negative." We are not here to discourage access to sexually oriented materials through the Internet. We do not promote censorship of any free medium of communication.

The purpose of this book and our work is to inform those who find their lives compromised by their repetitive patterns of sexual behavior that these issues can be treated and that help is available should they desire behavior change. To those whose lives have become caught up in a web of lies, self-deception, secrets, and isolation caused by compulsive sexual behaviors, we offer hope and opportunity to create change.

JENNIFER SCHNEIDER, M.D., Ph.D.
ROBERT WEISS, M.S.W., C.A.S.

Acknowledgments

The authors wish to thank the following colleagues for their help in making this book possible: Patrick Carnes, Al Cooper, Deborah Corley, David Delmonico, Michael Alvarez, John Sealy, Sharon O'Hara, Joyce Dohanian, Marnee Ferree, Bill Owen, Alex Katehakis, Reid Finlayson, Linda Hudson, Charlotte Kasl, Dana Putnam, Doug Weiss, Carol Ross, and Rich Salmon. We also gratefully acknowledge our supportive families, the help of our agent, Edite Kroll, and our editor, Corrine Casanova. Most of all, this book could not have happened without the many recovering people who put their trust in us and told us, often in detail, of how cybersex addiction had affected their lives.

ONE

Introduction to the World of Cybersex

◼ ◼ ◼

Jack, the oldest of four children, became the "man of the house" at age eleven, when his father left his mother for a younger woman. Jack's mother took on two jobs in order to feed the family, leaving Jack largely responsible for his three siblings. He shopped for their food, made sure they ate three meals a day, baby-sat them in the evenings, disciplined them when they misbehaved, and did more than his share of the housecleaning. Jack was very much "parentified," meaning that at times he was needed to be more the parent than the child. After college, Jack married Susanna, a very dependent young woman, and continued his pattern of feeling responsible for others' happiness. Several years after his wedding, he became involved with a secretary at work. The affair provided a haven from his responsibilities and gave him a chance to experience intrigue, excitement, and just plain fun, something with which he'd had very little experience. After a year, however, the secretary began pressuring Jack to leave his wife. When he refused, she told Susanna about the affair. Susanna's response was uncharacteristically independent: she divorced him.

When Jack got married for the second time, he told doubting buddies, "I mean it, this time no extramarital secret life." One wedding present, a home computer, gave Jack entry to a whole new world—the Internet. Unknown to his friends and new spouse, within six months of being married, Jack was involved nightly in three different online, or virtual, affairs, had downloaded more than 1,200 pornographic images, and was spending fifteen to twenty hours a week in sexual chat rooms and "membership clubs," trading and downloading new pictures—all of it a secret from his wife and accessed from his study at home.

Before their marriage, Jack and his second wife, Jody, had enjoyed an active and exciting sexual relationship, but gradually, as Jack's hidden Internet life became more arousing to him than sex with his wife, he grew more detached and withdrawn. Drawn to the computer whenever he was free at home, Jack began avoiding intimate moments with Jody. He would explain, "I'm so tired, but I still gotta go back into the study and get some work done tonight." After she was asleep, Jack would go into high gear, spending several hours in real-time interactive sexual activities with one or another of his favorite cybersex partners. With the help of electronic cameras hooked up to both their computers, he and his fantasy women could do everything sexually except actually touch each other. If one woman wasn't available, Jack would engage in sexual talk with another or else masturbate to the latest photos in his collection. In the early morning hours, Jack would slip into bed exhausted, awakened only a few hours later by the demands of his alarm clock. Another day had begun.

Like many businesses, Jack's office provided computers in each manager's office. When Jack was promoted to a managerial position, he acquired a private office and his own computer. At first on work breaks, and later increasing in frequency, he found that a brief, closed-door visit to an online porn site was more refreshing than a chat about sports with the salesmen. Jack justified his activities by telling himself, "I'm not actually cheating. I'm not having real sex with anyone else, and I'm not at risk for catching a sexually transmitted disease or exposing Jody to one. I'm just having some fun, and no one is being hurt." He told Jody that his heavy work schedule and new responsibilities were so draining that he was just not interested in sex for the time being.

For Jody, however, things had clearly changed from the close and exciting moments they had shared previously at the beginning of their relationship. At first, she was sympathetic to Jack. She knew he was working hard at his managerial job, she appreciated the extra income, and she convinced herself that the lack of intimacy was only temporary. Jody felt emotionally abandoned, but she persuaded herself that she was overreacting and that everything was fine. She threw herself harder into her own job as an accountant and gave Jack the space he needed. But one day, when she turned on the home computer to input the household expenses and write to an old friend, her whole world fell apart. Having unknowingly signed on with Jack's screen name, she was instantly assaulted by half a dozen disturbing e-mails:

- Wanna f##k me now?
- I am waiting to do it to you baby. . . .
- Sweetheart, why are you making me wait till tonight to curl up with you?

Shocked, but uncertain at first, Jody spent the next several hours at the computer discovering the trail of Jack's computer activities. She reviewed his online history, looked through his Internet address book, opened the hundreds of JPEG and GIF porn photo files, and read his previously sent and received e-mails. One letter contained plans for a rendezvous the following month at a nearby city where Jody knew that Jack would be attending a convention. Jody was devastated and wondered if she knew anything about the man she had married.

THE INTERNET REVOLUTION

New Opportunities and Conveniences

The Internet is profoundly transforming our culture and our world in ways similar to the introduction of the telephone in the early twentieth century. An interactive system connecting personal computers, the Internet was virtually unknown before 1993, when only a few people in laboratories, universities, and the U.S. government utilized it. Today, at the dawn of the twenty-first century, 55 percent of Americans have access to the Internet, and one-third of this group is online at least five hours a week.[1] The Internet has experienced a phenomenal growth. It offers an abundance of opportunities to learn and to meet people, offering information on almost any subject or question. The Internet provides rapid, inexpensive communication with people all over the world. The lonely business traveler no longer has to make costly phone calls home at odd hours. Travelers now send e-mail at their leisure, which recipients read at their convenience.

Time zones, distance, even national borders no longer hamper business dealings and friendships. Personal Web sites allow family members and friends around the world to instantly catch up on the latest news and baby pictures on the same medium as small shops in remote parts of the world display their products and wares. Personal letters or "snail mail" are rapidly vanishing from mailboxes, replaced by e-mail correspondence. And this is just the beginning.

Because of the Internet, access to up-to-the-minute information is no longer limited. People with chronic illnesses greet their doctors with computer printouts of the latest treatments for their medical problem. Online discussion groups allow free exchange of information and support for hundreds of medical conditions and personal concerns. Thousands of online chat groups and bulletin boards are geared toward every possible hobby, interest, and pursuit—from '50s automobiles to Zen Buddhist retreats. More people have access to more information than ever before. And they can find it on the computer screen—without leaving the safety net of home.

KEEPING UP WITH THE FAST PACE OF LIFE

Times are rapidly changing. Have you ever watched an old-time classic movie or read a nineteenth-century novel and been disappointed at the molasses-slow pace? Did you know that current television programs and movies now have shorter and more numerous scenes than programming of twenty years ago? The rapid scene changes of the MTV world are becoming our entertainment norm. Inexorably and without being aware of it, we have become accustomed to a much faster pace in many areas of our lives.

The Internet is a logical extension of this accelerating pace of life. A hundred years ago life was very different. A visit to a relative who lived ten miles away was a major trip. It required an entire weekend to get there, visit, and return. A one-week turnaround time in response to a letter was considered quick. News events in Europe took many days to be publicized in the United States. On April 15, 1912, when the "unsinkable" *Titanic* collided with an iceberg and sank in the Atlantic Ocean, it took days before most people in the United States were aware of this tragedy. Today, news of a commercial plane crash is widely disseminated throughout the world within minutes. Seventy years ago, phones altered our expectations of personal communication to a more rapid response time. The popularity of fax machines by the late 1980s resulted in the ability to transfer written documents long-distance within minutes. But even then, people still expected to be going to libraries to research information sources and to bookstores to buy books and magazines.

The Internet has increased our expectations even further. Why learn at the library when the Internet can provide instant answers to nearly any question? The culture has become increasingly time-sensitive, and many people are too busy to wait for anything. They want information at their fingertips without having to leave the house to get it. The Internet is there to satisfy the increasing need for quick answers, instant gratification, and immediate action. The price to be paid, however, may be a large-scale increase in isolation.

Without doubt, the Internet can be cited as the number one cultural phenomenon of our age. It is rapidly becoming the most important instrument of social change in the developed world. This conclusion is supported in a recent study that showed that "the nation's obsession with the Internet is causing many Americans to spend less time with friends and family, less time shopping in stores, and more time working at home after hours."[2] The study's principal investigator, Norman Nie, a political scientist at Stanford University, said: "When you spend your time on the Internet, you don't hear a human voice and you never get a hug. There are going to be millions of people with very minimal human interaction." Not surprisingly, people who use the Internet to obtain information have also found it to be an intense and easy way to get their sexual needs met.

SEX: NEW ADVENTURES
THROUGH THE INTERNET

The Internet is leading a revolution in the delivery of sex and sexual content. Long before the dawn of the written alphabet and the later development of printing, cave dwellers created erotic art with scribbled drawings on stone walls. While visual and written pornography go back for many hundreds of years, not until now has sexual imagery and the invitation to interact with it been so readily accessible and affordable.

Sex, sexuality, and sexual expression of every conceivable variety and type have evolved as a dominant area of content and interest on the Internet. There is even a new word in the English language for this phenomenon—*cybersex*. We can define *cybersex* as any form of sexual expression that is accessed through the computer or the Internet. This book examines problematic cybersexual behavior, but it also addresses the issues that can arise from online romantic relationships and online affairs.

Currently, more than 60 percent of all visits and commerce on the Internet involve a sexual purpose. In 1999, the 28,000 or so online adult Web sites grossed at least one billion dollars.[3] Without the fear of discovery or potential embarrassment of a face-to-face interaction, people are asking about, investigating, and exchanging information about the most intimate details of sexuality and relationships. For most of these visitors, the Internet provides a fascinating new venue for access to, learning about, and experiencing sex. For these people, computer sex is but one more way to enjoy life, much like an occasional exotic dessert. The variety and novelty of cybersex may lead some of these people to temporarily indulge in it, even to excess, but most soon return to their usual sexual activities, relegating Internet sexual exploration to an occasional dalliance.

For these particular cybersex adventurers, their new experiences online can provide them with added energy and enthusiasm for sex with self, spouse, or significant other. When asked, they will affirm that cybersex can be a hot, exciting, and playful distraction. A significant minority of men and women, however, for whom the ease of access, anonymity, and velocity of the online sexual material is problematic, getting hooked on cybersex can lead to loss of jobs and relationships, as well as health, legal, or other concerns.

TYPES OF CYBERSEX USERS

Based on the findings of Cooper and his colleagues,[4] cybersex users can be divided into three types, which are listed below, along with their chief characteristics:

1. Recreational or Nonpathological Users

These users are people who discover sex on the Internet, find it interesting or fun, and get involved for short periods of time but not to extremes. Ultimately they find it a playful distraction but not meaningful. The following is often true of this type of usage:

- Curiosity, novelty, education, or entertainment drive the online activity.
- Viewing is intermittent and occasional.
- Interest in cybersex is not sustained over time because of a lack of face-to-face interaction, the repetitive nature of the two-dimensional images, and the unreality of the activity.

2. At-risk Users

These users are people who are vulnerable to addictive distractions due to life stress or underlying unhappiness. They use the cybersex activity in addictive ways for periods of time as a means of coping, sometimes even to the point of having negative consequences. They will generally respond to the adverse consequences by adjusting or stopping their behaviors. Without the Internet, they might not have developed the sexual addiction problem. Characteristics of at-risk users include the following:

- minimal history of sexually addictive behaviors or problematic sexual history
- some predisposition for dealing with emotional discomfort through sexual means or impulsive sexual behavior
- use of online sexual stimulation as a means of achieving distraction from stress or extremes of mood
- use of cybersex to escape the emotions of severe life stresses (such as a death in family, financial problems, or the birth of the first child)
- use of cybersex to replace personal communication and support

3. Sexually Addicted Users

These users are people who become hooked on cybersex regardless of the consequences. They feel compelled to engage in computer-driven romantic or sexual activity to the detriment of their personal lives. They do not have the ability, on their own, to stop the addictive behavior patterns. Characteristics of sexually addicted users include the following:

- history of childhood abuse, trauma, or neglect (particularly if not acknowledged or understood)
- history of addictions in the family of origin
- history of intimacy problems and relationship concerns
- previously established pattern of using drugs, alcohol, or compulsive behaviors (including work) as a means of coping with stress or difficult feelings
- possible history of anxiety, depression, or other emotional challenges
- social or emotional isolation
- tendency to live a double life

CAUGHT IN THE NET

Readers who wonder whether their own involvement with cybersex might be compulsive are invited to look at the Cybersex Addiction Checklist in appendix 1 (pages 196–197).

A groundbreaking cybersex survey by Cooper and associates of 9,265 Internet users found that 8.5 percent were sexually compulsive or addictive.[5] These cybersex users spent at least eleven hours per week in online sexual pursuits. They were considered addicts because they generally denied they had a problem, made repeated efforts to decrease their online sexual activities, and continued going online despite poor academic or job performance, relationship difficulties, job loss, sexual harassment suits, arrests, failed relationships, or other adverse consequences.

Approximately 1 percent of the cybersex addicts in a follow-up analysis of the groundbreaking Cooper cybersex survey had a lengthy history of sexual obsessions and compulsions that long preceded their discovery of sex on the Internet.[6] This group of people was acting in sexually addictive ways even before the Internet came along. For them, the computer simply became another means of expressing their sex addiction.

For both the at-risk user and the previously sex-addicted man or woman, the availability of the Internet spells trouble. Following is the story of Hank, who paid a high price for his cybersex adventures:

Hank, a forty-six-year-old married man, began downloading and viewing pornography and erotic stories online from almost the first day he got his computer. Over time this advanced to nightly participation in sexually oriented chat rooms while masturbating to the images and explicit communication that other people would offer him online. Despite having no previous history of adultery, Hank planned and carried out two extramarital sexual encounters with long-term online sexual partners, seeking help only when his wife found out about his behavior. Hank writes of the many consequences of his cybersex involvement:

> Looking back, I am amazed by the immense amount of time and energy I put into my cybersex activity. It created emotional distance, frustration, and impatience in my relationships with my wife and children and took up work time and office resources. Eventually I was caught and nearly fired; I may yet be terminated for this. Staying up long past midnight nearly every night, usually getting only three to six hours of sleep, caused sleep deprivation, depression, and physical health consequences. My sex life with my wife became practically nonexistent, and I watched her blame herself for this. Money we didn't have was spent on pay-per-view porn sites and digital video camera computer equipment to access and engage in live online sex acts. I even bought gifts for some online sex partners whom I never even had met. My teenage son found my porn stash one day on the computer and began

"collecting" it for himself. He has caught me on more than one occasion viewing pornography. He knows it is wrong and that I am wrong to be involved with it. My son and I have kept the secret of our online porn use from his mother, my wife. If I lose my job over this addiction, the impact will be major—possible loss of our home, ruined finances, emotional turmoil in the family, and possible divorce. Yet still I think about getting back online all the time.

Rosalie is a married thirty-five-year-old systems analyst. Having made it through a rough and impoverished childhood, which she had decided to just "put behind her," she was pleased to finally be in a peaceful and stable family of her own. A mother of two children, she felt content with her life. This changed rapidly with her discovery of online sex:

One day at work I accidentally stumbled across a porn site by hitting the wrong key when I was looking for a business Web site on the computer. Curiosity is why I went back. Within a matter of days, I was visiting porn sites on a daily basis; within weeks it seems like that was all I did. It literally took control and consumed my life. I went from joining all the free stuff to accessing anything I could to fuel my interest. I didn't want to go home. I began to lie to my husband about having to work late just so I could continue. I lost my mind in such a short time that I could not function at work or home. It took all I could do to hold up a straight face among my co-workers and family. I became very withdrawn and depressed. My mind became filled with dark and hurtful images, including bestiality. I felt like such a bad person, but I didn't know who to turn to. I guess that cybersex can take some people down a road they never dreamed they would go. I somehow got sucked into it and it has been hell to get out.

THE LURE OF THE NET

Hank and Rosalie are examples of people who got quickly hooked on the Net. What is it about computer sex that can make it so powerful and addicting? Dr. Alvin Cooper, an expert on cybersex addiction, believes that the intensity and lure of the Internet are powered by "The Triple A Engine," that is, the accessibility, affordability, and anonymity of the Internet.

Accessibility

With computers finding their way into more and more homes each day, Internet access grows to millions and millions of people. An estimated nine to fifteen million people access the Internet daily, and this rate is estimated to be growing by up to 25 percent every three months.[7] Moreover, it no longer takes a genius to figure out how to access the Internet. Software, once an engineering mystery, is now easier to use. Icons on the screen and helpful prompts make use of the computer feasible even for very young children. Children are now learning how to operate computers in preschool. Computer games have made the computer into a toy suitable for three- and four-year-olds; a whole generation is growing up as comfortable with typing and with using the computer as their parents were at their age in using the telephone. The Internet is very, very accessible.

Affordability

In the 1970s, computers were prohibitively expensive, occupied large rooms, and were truly functional only for government and large corporate use. Today, much more powerful computers take up no more than a corner of a desk, are relatively inexpensive, and cost almost nothing to use. An evening spent in a pornographic bookstore or strip club might cost hundreds of dollars, whereas an evening spent on the computer might cost forty cents. Unlimited Internet access is available for less than twenty dollars per month. The Internet has made entertainment in general, and sexual entertainment in particular, more affordable than ever before.

Anonymity

As a long-distance medium of communication, the Internet has many possibilities that person-to-person contact does not. It allows the user to try out different roles, to assume any identity or any characteristics he or she wishes: A five-foot-four-inch, fifty-year-old man weighing in at three hundred pounds can present himself in a teenage chat room as an eighteen-year-old high school basketball player, or as a sixteen-year-old girl looking for a pen pal. Most people who visit chat rooms change some facts about themselves, often their age, physical appearance, even their gender. In the recent Cooper survey of more than nine thousand Internet users, 48 percent reported that they changed their age "occasionally," and 23 percent reported they did so "often." Thirty-eight percent of the entire sample reported changing their race while online; 5 percent admitted to occasionally claiming to be the opposite sex, or "gender bending."[8]

Many people use false names, or "handles," to increase their anonymity. The Internet by nature is very anonymous. Online users have a perception of complete privacy in their interactions. Not having to leave home eliminates the possibility of being observed or caught by a neighbor, friend, or co-worker somewhere in the midst of a sexual interaction (with a prostitute, in a massage parlor or public park). Users can access desirable Web sites right from their own living room or bedroom. People who would be embarrassed to be caught sitting in a pornographic movie house or lurking in a porno bookstore welcome the opportunity to do these same activities in the privacy of their home (or—all too often—in their office at work).

The accessibility, affordability, and anonymity of online use make it very attractive, particularly for sexual intrigue. Other features that increase the lure of the Internet for cybersex users follow:

Secrecy

For someone wanting to keep a sexual secret, the problem with bringing a pornographic magazine or video home is that during or after the activity, the physical evidence remains. This makes it harder to keep the activity a secret from significant others or children. The computer, on the other hand, leaves no obvious traces. If an unwanted visitor enters the room, a flick of a finger changes the screen on the computer, and the user can feign innocence. (Many cybersex users are unaware that a history of computer activities remains automatically stored on the computer hard drive, even when "deleted," although it takes some computer savvy on the part of the "detective" to find the evidence).

Safety

The computer permits the user to engage in real-time online sex with another person—but without the risk of catching a sexually transmitted disease (STD), getting embroiled in an illegal financial exchange (with a prostitute or in a massage parlor), or getting arrested (for public or anonymous sex).

Normalization

On the Internet, users can find support for any type of sexual behavior, meeting other individuals with similar proclivities.

Within the framework of anonymity and privacy, users who have unusual or unconventional sexual interests—such as those with paraphilias (unhealthy, sometimes illegal sexual problems) or those with healthy but culturally frowned upon lifestyles (gays and lesbians, those interested in transvestitism or dominance-based sex)—can find other like-minded people who share and support these behaviors and who are willing to engage in them. This constant support and reinforcement of a particular behavior can validate the activity. It is easier and safer to interact with such people online than in person. Not surprisingly, Internet users with similar unconventional sexual interests have formed "virtual communities" for sexual activities and support of their sexual lifestyles.

SEXUAL ACTIVITIES AVAILABLE ON THE INTERNET

Those who are not familiar with the Internet may be surprised to learn that online sexual activity goes far beyond simply viewing pornography (cyberporn). Here are some other online activities:

- downloading and printing out pornographic images or saving them on a hard drive
- joining sexual paid-subscription membership communities that serve various sexual interests
- posting personal sex ads and then meeting people for sexual talk and/or sexual activities online or in person
- joining chat rooms or entering private chats, where people type real-time conversations (cyber-chat) back and forth to each other
- meeting a group of people who have similar interests (examples include "women having affairs," "spouses—

up after dark," "she/males tonight") through the use of chats or newsgroups
- exchanging e-mails and photos with others for the purpose of gathering phone numbers, arranging meetings, or engaging in relating fantasies or sexual talk
- online viewing of traditional (print or film) sex-industry products such as magazines and videos.
- participating in simultaneous mutual sexual activities with another person through a private chat room or a phone call and/or exchanging real-time digital photographs and video, transmitted through electronic digital cameras hooked up to the users' computers
- finding various sexually oriented newsgroups, which, like Web sites and chat rooms, are a way to access porn materials and sexual messages from others.

Newsgroups are posted on servers throughout the Internet on almost every subject from lawn care to German shepherds and are basically lists of messages and downloads like a bulletin board. Newsgroups are hard to monitor and police as they often are moved from one online address to another, particularly the more illicit ones. Sexually oriented newsgroups are often monitored by U.S. federal agencies in an attempt to capture those involved in the inappropriate exchange of materials.

CYBERSEX ACTIVITIES MAKE THE HEADLINES

Jack, whose story begins this chapter, agreed to attend counseling when his cybersex addiction resulted in his marriage crisis. At that time, he was only beginning to access sexually explicit Internet sites at work. Had his boss caught him participating in cybersex at work, he might have lost his job. Here are some news accounts of people who have had public consequences due to their online sexual interactions:

◘ Stamford, Connecticut, October 1999: Xerox Corporation, the world's biggest copier maker, said Wednesday it has fired more than twenty employees so far this year for looking at pornographic Internet sites at work. In total, forty Xerox employees have been fired this year for inappropriate use of the Internet, half of the firings related to pornography use.[9]

◘ Boston, Massachusetts, May 1999: Computer Porn Undoes a Divinity-school Dean: When Ronald Thiemann asked his university tech-support team to upgrade his hard drive last fall, it seemed like a routine request to turbo-charge a data-clogged computer. But the operation proved anything but routine. A techie's curious eye caught sight of an extensive collection of hard-core pornography. *The Boston Globe* later reported that Thiemann, dean of Harvard's Divinity School, had lost his post over porn.[10]

◘ Kennebunkport, Maine, October 1998. Retired Air Force pilot Kenneth Nighbert flew his American flag upside down from his second-floor sun deck, a universal cry for help. Then he went inside, tied a plastic bag around his head, and died. The event that caused him to asphyxiate himself took place on September 3, when he was snared in a fourteen-nation raid on an Internet pornography ring made up of people who allegedly were producing, selling, trading, and, in Nighbert's case, downloading pictures of little kids having sex. . . . A dozen people accused of being pedophiles killed themselves during a big Internet porn sweep two years ago in Belgium and France.[11]

▣ San Francisco, California, August 24, 1999: In what health officials believe is the first time a disease cluster has been traced to cyberspace, the department of public health here has tracked an outbreak of syphilis cases to an America Online chat room. Officials from the San Francisco Department of Public Health said six men who had contracted syphilis in the last three months have traced their last sexual encounters to partners they met through a chat room. These men represent a sizable number of the seventeen syphilis cases reported in San Francisco this year, and the cluster has provided a frightening glimpse of a potentially larger public health risk, as more and more people use computers to find sex partners, officials said.[12]

CYBERSEX: SIMPLY FUN, OR ADDICTIVE?

These stories likely represent the tip of the iceberg. Every day more people access Internet sexual sites, and some of them suffer negative consequences. Yet for many others, the Internet in general, and the Internet's sex sites in particular, are great sources of pleasure and contain information that enhances their lives. When are cybersex activities simply fun, and when are they addictive?

Consider David, a divorced fifty-eight-year-old man, now several years into attempted recovery from a sexual addiction, which began when he was thirteen years old. For several years before he found help, while he was still married, David's addiction took the form of Internet surfing, looking for pornography in newsgroups, downloading thousands of images, participating in sexually oriented newsgroups, and engaging in fantasy sex play online:

My constantly being on the computer took me away from business. My sex life has always been one of fantasy. I used to say to myself, "Hey, what's the big deal—I look at porn, masturbate, who's getting harmed? No one." Nothing could have been more untrue! After being on the Net and using porn, normal sex was totally unfulfilling and there wasn't a closeness or intimacy with my partner. I also isolated myself from my grown children and do not have a healthy relationship with them.

Cybersex addiction doesn't just come from having a computer or access to the Web. In my experience cybersex addiction comes from the *ease* with which a person who already has a sex addiction problem can access anything and everything sexual that one can imagine. On the Internet, sex addicts can use the largest porn shop in the world without leaving their offices or homes. There is almost total safety, as no one is going to see you there. It's cheap, and a huge amount is free for the taking. It's convenient; you can go there twenty-four hours a day and stay as long as you choose. It can and will feed *any* fantasy, some that you didn't even know existed.

My cybersex addiction has destroyed any real intimacy with the opposite sex and my marriage of twenty-five years. It has caused me to isolate myself from my friends and family. It has helped to further deteriorate an already poor sense of self-esteem and has deepened my depression and at times led to thoughts of suicide. Cybersex has played a real role in bringing me the most depraved thoughts and images that one could imagine. This is truly insanity for me.

INTERNET ADDICTION

In her book *Caught in the Net,* Dr. Kimberly S. Young wrote in detail about the problems families have when living with a person whose major preoccupation is computer games, chatting with friends online, or surfing the Net.[13] In such families, the partner feels lonely, ignored, unimportant, neglected, or angry because the Internet user prefers to spend so much time glued to the computer. In addition, children are neglected or ignored because of the parent's Internet involvement. Some Internet users are clearly hooked on the Net—that is, they are compulsive users, they continue their Internet activities despite significant adverse consequences, and they spend a great deal of time either involved in Internet activities or thinking about their past or future Internet activities. When they sit down in front of the computer, they may plan to spend only an hour or so there, but somehow time just slips by while they are engrossed in their online activities. They cannot reliably predict how much time they will actually spend on the Internet. They have, in fact, lost control of their Internet activities. Loss of control is a key element in any addiction.

CHARACTERISTICS OF AN ADDICT

As we will see in the next chapter, behaviors as well as substances can become compulsive or addictive. With alcohol, addiction is not defined by the number of drinks consumed but rather the consequences that alcohol use has on your life. A person can be considered an addict when all three of the following are present:

- when the person has lost control of the frequency of his or her engagement in an activity and participates in it compulsively
- when the behavior is continued despite significant negative consequences to the person in terms of his or her relationships, job, or health

- when the person spends a great deal of time preoccupied with the activity

As Young points out, more and more people are becoming addicted to Internet activities.

THE CONSEQUENCES

Any kind of sexual activity can become obsessive and can be used in an addictive manner, but the accessibility, affordability, and anonymity of the Internet make online sex a particularly enticing addictive experience. Compulsive use of online sex creates specific consequences that go beyond compulsive use of the Internet in general. These problems, affecting significant others, families, and children, result specifically from the sexual content of the user's Internet addiction. Here are some warning signs of Internet addiction:

- isolation from dating, social interaction, and the potential to meet available romantic partners (single people)
- reduction in spousal intimacy, sexuality, and communication (married people and those in committed relationships)
- increased guilt and shame about covering up the cybersex activities
- repeated lies and justifications about online sexual activities, and repeated promises to stop or change
- mistrust and betrayal
- potential job loss—more likely for cybersex activities at work than for nonsexual workplace online use
- contracting a sexually transmitted disease from real-life physical contact with cybersex partners and risking infecting a spouse or partner

- loss of self-esteem and self-worth by spouses/partners trying to "measure up" to a fantasy online lover
- children exposed to pornography when they accidentally step into the room when a parent is involved in cybersex activities or when they later find pornography on the computer
- children ignored or emotionally neglected due to a parent's obsession with having the time and ability to engage in online sex

Although the Internet can enhance the lives of most of its users, the obsessive and compulsive use of cybersex can destroy the lives of those caught in its grip. In upcoming chapters, we will describe in greater detail what constitutes an addiction, the features of sex addiction in general, the characteristics that make a person vulnerable to addiction, and what life is like for a person obsessed with cybersex. We will then look at the world of the woman who is addicted to cybersex and cyber-romance, and then at the perspective of spouses or partners of cybersex addicts. Subsequent chapters will describe how to get help and how to recover from the compulsive use of cybersex.

TWO

When Too Much Sex Is Not Enough

◙   ◙   ◙

Addiction is a concept that many people have trouble understanding. To a nonaddict, it seems inconceivable that a person would drink, use drugs, or engage in some addictive behavior to the point of serious consequences, unless that person had some moral flaw or weakness of character. Our Western culture of self-determination encourages the belief that those challenged by their circumstances will "just pull themselves up by the bootstraps" or "do the right thing." Others believe that calling oneself an "addict" is really just seeking an excuse to write off "bad behavior" and avoid facing up to one's problems. These notions are magnified in the area of addictive sexual behavior, where blaming problem sexual behavior on one's "sex addiction" might appear as an attractive alternative to taking responsibility.

THE NEUROCHEMISTRY OF ADDICTION

When people are under the influence of alcohol or drugs, perceptions change, moods shift, and attitudes and intentions are altered by the use of the substance. Some people engage in sexual activities they would not do while sober; others abuse their spouse or partner; still others drive their vehicle recklessly or attempt to become the life of the party. These changes in behavior can be attributed to the effect alcohol or drug consumption has on the brain. While some people use their consumption of alcohol or other drugs as an excuse for behaviors they would have liked to engage in anyway, these chemicals do indeed affect the brain, and some people become addicted.

It is often easier to understand addiction to a substance than to a behavior. The reality is that arousing or stimulating activities can be highly addictive for some according to how it affects their brain chemistry. Whereas drug and alcohol addictions can be defined as "a problematic relationship to a mood-altering *substance*," sex addiction can be defined as "a problematic relationship to a mood-altering *experience*."[1] For the cybersex addict, experiencing the intensity, excitement, and arousal of watching online pornography, hanging out in sexual chat rooms, or engaging in online video feeds becomes increasingly more important over time than other priorities or relationships. Similar to the drug addict, the sex addict becomes less and less interested in the real relationships and experiences that make up a healthy life.

Questions about Behavior Addictions

- How do these experiences become addictive?
- How can someone become addicted to a behavior?
- How can gambling, sex, or risk-taking behaviors actually become addictive to the point of hooking someone?

The answers to these questions lie in the neurochemistry of addiction: People can become addicted to a behavior when it causes chemical changes in the brain that are intense, powerful, and arousing to them. They then become addicted to the way their behaviors can influence their own neurochemistry. These powerful self-produced chemicals such as adrenaline (epinephrine), serotonin, dopamine, and endorphins create a distracting and intense druglike state for behavioral addicts. People become addicted to the behaviors that cause intense changes in the body. In reality, people addicted to sex, gambling, and compulsive spending *are* drug addicted. They have just found a way to induce the chemical release within their own system, rather than introducing an external source. People who are addicted to sex, gambling, food, high-risk taking, overspending, and so on, are in fact addicted to mood/mind-altering experiences.

I Just Like to Party: Sam's Story

Sam, a twenty-eight-year-old single man, works as a clerk in his local bank. Although he devotes most weekends and money he can't afford partying on crack cocaine, he wouldn't describe himself as addicted. He says, "I just like to party." Though his finances are in shambles and his girlfriend has threatened to leave him unless he starts spending more time with her, he continues to spend two to three weekends a month smoking drugs at his dealer's house. Sam tells the story this way:

> A typical Friday before a partying weekend looks like this: When I get to work on Friday morning, I plan to spend the evening at home. For some reason, usually after lunch, I start thinking about going to see Fred (my drug dealer). I call him from work to see if he has any coke and whether there is going to be any partying at his house this weekend. If he says yes, I feel a jolt and I know I am going to participate. I begin preparations by withdrawing the cash I will need for the weekend. I leave work early, getting someone to spot for me. Driving downtown toward Fred's house, I start thinking about what it

will be like when I get there—the girls, the smoke, the party. I remember the hot times I had the last time I hung out there.

After parking my car, I walk up to the door and use that special knock; I can hear music and laughter inside. As soon as I arrive, I can already smell the drugs. It's exciting to run into a few girls I have had sex with before. Fred comes up with some coke in a pipe and asks me if I want to try it out before I buy. I sit down with him as he places the pipe in my mouth and lights it. I draw in a long, deep breath, taking my first hit of coke.

In reading the story above, ask yourself, At what point is Sam high? Is he high before he inhales the first hit of cocaine? In reality, Sam's body chemistry begins to change when he first thinks about getting high. This feeling escalates the closer he gets to his dealer's house. With each passing moment, Sam becomes more aroused by the thought of getting and using the drugs. When he first muses about it in the office, Sam's heart begins to race as his drug-related fantasies cause adrenaline to release in his body. His entire body reacts: pupils dilate, hands become clammy, hearing becomes more acute, and breathing becomes more rapid and shallow. Sam enters a mildly altered physiological state of arousal that becomes more intense as he gets closer to the object of his fantasy, the dealer's house and the drugs. Thoughts about finances or his girlfriend are banished by the intense arousal he is feeling. Once inside the dealer's house, Sam reels with the excitement of anticipation: physically and emotionally he is ready for that first hit of coke.

Sam is high long before he inhales the first hit of cocaine at his dealer's house. Addiction specialists understand that Sam's own psychobiological arousal system kicked in at his earliest thoughts of using. Each step in Sam's travels brought him more and more into arousal, distraction, and fantasy, thereby increasing production of the neurochemicals of arousal. The arousal process and the self-induced euphoria it created left Sam less and less able to make good, healthy choices for himself. If one believed that euphoria could occur only when using a drug, then Sam could not have been high until he put the pipe to his mouth and smoked. Yet if that were the case, how can the strong changes in his thinking and body chemistry prior to the drug use be explained?

Understanding Sex Addiction

Imagining the euphoric feelings created by the thoughts, fantasies, and planning of behaviors helps us better understand the nature of sex addiction.

When sitting in front of the computer, waiting for the chosen images of cyberporn or sexual chats to download, cybersex addicts are already high. They are in a state of self-induced neurochemical intensity, rendering themselves relatively powerless to change their behaviors or to consider how their behaviors affect others in the long term. People in treatment for various addictions often call this state "the trance" or "being in the bubble." It is the same arousal state that allows compulsive gamblers to bet away their homes or children's college funds. It's the same fantasy-fueled intensity that can keep a sex addict compulsively cruising a particular street for hours seeking prostitutes. Psychologists compare this self-induced state to a "fight-or-flight" or "survival mode." It is actually a useful and necessary state a person enters when a crisis or threat requires the person's complete focus, intention, and readiness. The phenomenon of "fight-or-flight arousal" is demonstrated below:

Mary, a five-foot-four-inch, 124-pound woman walks down the street with her seven-year-old son toward the grocery store. Distracted by her shopping list, she doesn't notice when her son runs out into the street after a puppy. Rushing head-long into the street without looking, her son is hit by a passing compact car and falls near the sidewalk. Conscious, but pinned beneath the car, the boy is unable to free himself. Instantly jolted with panic, Mary runs over to her son and, in a moment of terror-based intensity, lifts up the car by its bumper with her right hand and pulls her son free with her left.

How is this possible? How did this 124-pound woman lift up a 1,800-pound car? Was this a conscious act? Did she plan to cross the street and lift up that car? If you had asked her a few moments before the accident occurred, "Excuse me, ma'am, could you please cross the street and lift up that VW bug for a minute or two?" she would have laughed out loud. In truth, during moments of fear, excitement, and intensity, we can use the physical state induced by our own body chem-istry to engage our strength for survival. But in those mo-ments, part of what this rush of chemicals does is block out our conscious, rational, intellectual thought process. Mary wasn't thinking about moving that car; she just did it. A part of the syndrome of fight-or-flight is that the adrenaline, en-dorphins, and other brain chemicals being produced help us address the immediate crisis moment by narrowing our thought process. We are literally not thinking, but acting com-pletely in the present. The description above may help to un-derstand the type of arousal/intensity state that is mirrored in a cybersex addict's behavior.

Locked into fantasy and obsession as the person spends hours online, the sex addict's physiologically euphoric state is maintained by the ongoing chatting, searching, and down-loading of images and experiences. This activity keeps him or her distracted and literally not thinking of other priorities, relationships, or experiences. When a spouse confronts the addict and says, "What about me and our relationship? Didn't you think about how your looking at the porn every night was affecting us?" the cybersex addict will answer in the negative, admitting that he or she was totally focused on the computer screen and the immediate moment. Cybersex addicts will sit in front of their computers, even saying to themselves, "I'll stop in ten minutes, I'll stop for dinner, I'll stop to put the kids to bed. . . ." Often, ten minutes becomes two or three hours. Dinner gets cold, and frustrated loved ones give up waiting and go to bed.

For the cybersex addict and sex addicts in general, the goal of all the looking, cruising, contacting, and downloading is not necessarily the orgasm. In fact, orgasm is not always a welcome or desired part of the process. Most porn and cybersex addicts look at images or remain in sexual chat for hours on end, maintaining the desired level of self-stimulation—but once orgasm occurs, the game is over and reality floods in. At this point, the addict is reminded of the late hour, the promises made and broken, and yet another night of not enough sleep. Interestingly, the goal of cybersex isn't orgasm; it is to maintain the hyperarousal state for as long as possible, returning again and again to the euphoria and intensity provided by an unending stream of images, words, and interaction on the Internet.

CHARACTERISTICS OF ADDICTION

Think of the people you know who like to drink alcohol. What characteristics separate social or occasional drinkers from alcoholics? Is it how many beers they drink in one evening? The time they spend in bars? How do you decide? Addiction specialists say that addiction is not defined by the number of drinks a person consumed, but rather the effect of the drinking on that person's life.

All addictions, whether to alcohol, drugs, gambling, or online sexual addiction, are characterized by the following three elements, all of which must be present in order to define the problem as an addiction:

1. Loss of control over the behavior (for example, drinking, eating, surfing the Net): The behavior has become compulsive and the person has lost the ability to stop when he or she wishes.
2. Continuation despite adverse consequences: These may include relationship problems, job loss, health problems, or legal concerns.
3. Preoccupation or obsession: Spending large amounts of time thinking about the activity or being actively involved in it.

It is crucial to understand that for any addiction, what matters is not the quantity of the behavior (or the number of drinks), but rather the consequences of that set of behaviors on a person's life. When all three of the above criteria are met, then a person can be said to be truly addicted to that activity. (If only one or two criteria are present, the person may be said to be "abusing" the drug or behavior, or has a problem with it, or is "at risk" of addiction, but is not necessarily addicted.) Viewed in this light, some people can be termed "Internet addicts," while others, whom we will call "cybersex addicts," are addicted to specific activities on the Internet, such as viewing sexual content or engaging in romantic or sexual chats.

Another typical characteristic of addiction is tolerance—needing more and more of the drug or behavior to get the same effect. Alcoholics often find themselves drinking more liquor to feel the same euphoria that a small amount initially induced. Pathological gamblers usually find themselves betting larger and larger amounts of money more often. As the addictive behavior escalates, so do the adverse consequences.

ADDICTION IS A RELATIONSHIP

Although many people find it hard to understand behavior addictions such as compulsive cybersex, they have no difficulty intuitively understanding addiction to alcohol or another drug. Even some professionals in the addiction field mistakenly assume that what causes an addiction is a drug entering the body and changing the brain chemistry. The reality is that addiction is a *relationship*—an intimate and overpowering connection between a person and a substance or an activity.

To begin to understand this, imagine a change of scene—the neighborhood bar instead of the den at home, and a drink in hand instead of the computer mouse. Joe stops at the bar on the way home, intending to have a drink or two and be home in time for dinner. Instead, Joe ends up spending three or four hours there, having six or eight beers, and returns home too late even to kiss his children good night. Joe's wife is furious, and Joe apologizes and promises to be on time the next day. Only two days later, the same scenario is replayed. As it becomes clear that Joe places a higher priority on drinking than on his family life, his spouse begins to feel lonely, ignored, unimportant, neglected, and angry. Notice that it is the relationship to the substance that causes Joe the problem, not the use of the substance itself. Many people enjoy alcohol or even recreational drugs without experiencing any long-term consequences or ill effects. Healthy people are able to engage with potentially addictive substances and experiences, while keeping their priorities straight. Yet people who are addicts get into trouble because they become increasingly invested in preserving their relationship with the drug, to the exclusion of other relationships. Work, significant others, family, and children become less and less important than having access to and using alcohol. The same misalignment of priorities takes place for cybersex addicts who increasingly lose sight of their life goals while becoming more and more engaged in their on-line activity.

People who are addicted to substances and behaviors lose the ability to see reality clearly. They give up their most important life relationship—the one with themselves. The rational and self-reflective relationship with self that allows healthy people to make good choices is gradually replaced by the relationship with the drug or intensity-inducing behavior; eventually the addict is completely out of touch with healthy reality. This separation from reality—maintained through denial, rationalization, blaming others, and justification—prevents the addict from seeing the results, outcome, or consequences of his or her behaviors. Loved ones are hurt, finances are ruined, jobs or even lives are lost, but the addict does not see himself or herself as responsible. In the end, the only relationship to which the addict holds any real allegiance is the drug or activity.

The real question is, Why would someone give up his or her relationship to reality for a drug? What does a mind-altering chemical or intensity-based experience offer someone that would be worth giving up his or her mental health to obtain? The answer is both obvious and complex. Addicts willingly give up reality in exchange for the ability to alter their mood at will. People who become addicted to substances and behaviors are people who have difficulty tolerating their own feelings and reactions. Irritability, anxiety, stress, embarrassment—even joy—are at times intolerable emotional experiences for addicts.

Drugs, alcohol, and intensity-based behaviors (such as sexual acting out, gambling, or risktaking) provide the means to tolerate and get through the challenges of emotional discomfort. The classic example of the shy person who can become the life of the party after a few drinks demonstrates clearly how substances allow addicts to more comfortably manage circumstances that they might otherwise find difficult. Addictive behaviors serve as a crutch for people who have not learned how to independently manage and cope with their own moods and feelings. This may stem from hereditary or childhood environments—most likely from both. For addicts, abuse or dependency upon substances or behaviors is a logical and adaptive tool for managing uncomfortable and sometimes chaotic emotional states. This tool can be replaced only by proper redirection, support, and the gradual introduction of new coping skills.

TYPES OF ADDICTIVE SEXUAL BEHAVIORS

In his 1983 book, *Out of the Shadows: Understanding Sexual Addiction*, Dr. Patrick Carnes categorized problematic sexual behaviors into three levels, based on the way society views them legally and ethically.[2]

◼ Level One—Sexual behaviors that have the potential to become addictive but are generally acceptable. These include masturbation, straight or gay sexual relations with multiple partners, pornography, cybersex use, and some forms of prostitution. These behaviors enhance the lives of most people, causing problems only if they become excessive or unmanageable. Most people who engage in these kinds of sexual activities enjoy them and are not troubled by the outcome or results.

(Prostitution is a special case because it is illegal in most places in the United States and thus can cause the consumer legal problems if caught.)

◉ Level Two—Sexual behaviors that are considered nuisance crimes, therefore falling out of the boundaries of acceptable behaviors. These include exhibitionism, voyeurism, public sex (in beaches, parks, and so on), anonymous sex, obscene phone calls, and *frotteurism* (touching another person without permission). Most people who are arrested for these activities have a long history of such behaviors, often with previous arrests. Many people who break laws to have sex or "casually" sexually offend are sexually addicted. Some are simply sex offenders and may or may not have addictive patterns.

◉ Level Three—Sexual behaviors that are more serious crimes. These include rape, child molestation, obtaining and using child pornography, sexual abuse of older adults, and incest.

Cybersex addiction can be found in each of Carnes's three levels. Viewing Internet pornography and engaging in real-time cybersex with unknown sexual partners are level one behaviors. The recent practices of illicitly videotaping nude athletes in locker rooms and surreptitiously videotaping up women's dresses while standing in line behind them ("upskirting")—and then transmitting such tapes on the Internet—are examples of level two behaviors. Soliciting child pornography online or seeking children for sex through the Internet are level three behaviors. The technology is the only thing new about these activities.

SEX ADDICT VERSUS SEX OFFENDER

Because Carnes's classification emphasized the law, this is a good place to clarify the distinction between sex addict and sex offender. To review, a *sex addict* is a person who engages compulsively in one or more sexual behaviors, who continues the behaviors despite significant negative consequences, and who spends a great deal of time thinking about the sexual activities. A *sex offender* is a person whose sexual behavior has broken the law, often by violating another person. Law-abiding sex addicts may lose their health, marriage, or job, but they are not sex offenders. Many sex offenders are not sex addicts. For example, most rapists rape out of anger or out of a desire to obtain power over their victims or to hurt their victims; very few rapists are sexually addicted. Geral T. Blanchard found that 55 percent of 109 imprisoned sex offenders were sexually addicted, including 71 percent of child molesters and 39 percent of men convicted of adult rapes.[3] Richard Irons and Jennifer Schneider found that among approximately two hundred physicians and therapists who sexually exploited their patients (an illegal behavior that defined all these professionals as sex offenders), about 55 percent were sexually addicted.[4]

Earlier in this chapter, tolerance and escalation of the behavior as aspects of addiction were discussed. Some readers of Carnes's book misunderstood his grouping to suggest that tolerance in sex addiction meant that with time, sex addicts progressed from harmless to dangerous behaviors, from legal to illegal activities. Worried spouses would ask, "If my husband masturbates compulsively, should I worry about him eventually molesting our children?"

Although exhibitionists and child molesters often engage in pornography and masturbation, which are level one behaviors, most level one sex addicts do not engage in level two or three behaviors. They are more likely to intensify their level one behaviors. For example, a cybersex addict who begins by viewing pornography on the Internet may progress to spending more time at sexually oriented Internet sites, then to having online real-time sexual encounters, and subsequently meeting these partners in person. But all these behaviors remain within level one.

SEXUAL ADDICTION: A PROBLEM FOR MEN *AND* WOMEN

Although many assume that sex addiction is primarily a problem for men, approximately 25 percent of the members of Twelve Step recovery programs for sexual addiction are women. Despite a lot of overlap, women's sex addiction tends to take somewhat different patterns from that of men: Women are more likely to get into fantasy relationships and to exhibit their bodies (using seductive clothing, for example), and less likely to have anonymous sex partners or to spend a lot of time viewing pornography.

Recent research compares the way women and men use the Internet for sex. In Cooper's survey of more than nine thousand Internet users, women constituted 14 percent of the entire group. However, they constituted 21 percent of cybersex addicts.[5] In other words, although most Internet users in Cooper's study were men, women were overrepresented among cybersex addicts relative to nonaddicts who use the Internet. One hypothesis, according to Cooper, is that women who use the Internet are more at risk of developing sexual compulsions. Another possibility, however, is that women may be less prone than men to deny that they have a problem, since it is less acceptable for a female in our society to use the computer for sexual pursuits.

Women's online sexual activities also differ from those of men. Women tend to prefer chat rooms to other mediums and use the Web less often for sexual pursuits. Men have the opposite pattern: they prefer the Web and use chat rooms as their second choice for engaging in sexual activities.[6] This supports women's preference for sex within the context of a relationship, whereas men seem more comfortable with anonymous or objectified sex.

Many women do fall into patterns of sexual acting-out behaviors that prove to be both intense and self-destructive. Consider the case of Joyce:

> For many years, Joyce, a thirty-four-year-old married accountant and mother of three children, had been an avid consumer of television soap operas and romance novels. These stories would transport her from her mundane existence to a romantic, exciting world of endless bliss in exotic locations. Though she had not had an affair, she frequently masturbated to fantasies related to co-workers, family friends, and the fantasy characters in her television shows. When Roy, Joyce's husband, an engineer, bought a computer for their home, she initially used it to maintain the household bills while using e-mail to contact family and friends.
>
> While scanning the Internet one day, Joyce entered the world of Internet chat rooms, quickly finding herself spellbound by the exciting men and personal conversations she encountered there. Within weeks, Joyce was staying up long after Roy was asleep, chatting with other "marrieds" about their lives and personal situations. Conversations in open chat rooms led to regular online "meetings" with specific men with whom she felt particularly comfortable.
>
> Over several weeks these interactions became increasingly more intimate, personal, and sexual in nature. Joyce began to

feel more fully understood and connected to these men than to her own husband, who in comparison seemed too dull, needy, and demanding. Nights on the computer gradually became Joyce's primary source of excitement and distraction, as they began to include masturbation and sexual chat. In the morning, she'd drag herself off to work, and by evening she was often too tired to even help with family meals. She frequently nodded off for a couple of hours in front of the TV after dinner. But when her husband went to sleep, Joyce came to life again on the computer. Roy, thinking that Joyce was ill or stressed out, kept suggesting she take some time off from work or see a doctor to find out why she was so tired and why she had lost interest in their lovemaking. Joyce said it was the busy tax season at work so she couldn't take time off, and although she agreed to make an appointment with her doctor, she somehow never got around to it.

Joyce never let on about her nightly liaisons, believing them to be a personal fantasy, unrelated to her marital relationship, just like the romance novels had been. In time, one of Joyce's online chat partners mentioned that he was going on a business trip to her city and suggested an offline meeting. Filled with a mixture of fear and excitement, Joyce met and had sex with this man at his hotel. Her addictive behavior rapidly escalated into a pattern of having sexual chats and masturbation with more men online, which led to sexual encounters with several of those partners offline. Joyce's secret fantasy life came to a crashing halt several months later when her husband confronted her after he caught a sexually transmitted disease from her.

Joyce was a cybersex user who became addicted to the intense arousal she experienced in her fantasy life.

Her story did not have a happy ending: Her husband of fourteen years, feeling betrayed and outraged, filed for divorce. After nearly losing custody of her three children, Joyce finally sought help and began the lengthy process of rebuilding her shattered life.

Without recovery, all addictions continue despite adverse consequences. Only when the consequences are severe enough does the addict usually seek help. This stage is often referred to as "bottoming out." Each type of addiction has its own particular consequences. The losses that pathological gamblers experience typically are financial. Alcoholics experience many health consequences, even before they have problems in their relationships or jobs. The consequences experienced by cyber-sex addicts are more clearly defined in the following chapter.

THREE

Cybersex Out of Control

◨ ◨ ◨

Alan, a thirty-eight-year-old investment counselor with a large international firm, considered himself a longtime "porn fan." Alan's father had always been an avid consumer of pornography, and as Alan got into his teens, his illicit peeks into his father's magazines were replaced with a burgeoning collection of his own. Later, Alan supplemented the printed material with a substantial number of porn videotapes, which he enjoyed viewing while masturbating. When he was in his twenties and actively dating, Alan continued masturbating at least daily. He considered himself a man with a high sex drive and nothing more.

At age thirty, Alan became engaged to Penny, a personal fitness trainer, with whom he had an active and enjoyable sexual relationship. When Penny moved into Alan's apartment, she was dismayed and upset to discover his extensive pornography collection and persuaded him to discard all the magazines and videos. Around the time of their marriage, Alan got a new job with a prestigious company and became very involved with his career. Over the next seven years, with his demanding job and Penny's increasing responsibilities at home with their young child as well as her active career, their sex life lost some of its excitement. However, Alan considered his life to be good.

One day, while using the Internet at work, Alan came upon

an online pornography site. The thrill he experienced reminded him of his long-discarded porn and brought back memories of the exciting sex he used to have. He felt like a "kid in a candy store" and eagerly sought more. Over the next few weeks, he returned to the frequent masturbation habit of his past, which quickly became a secret from his wife. Whereas sex with Penny had become routine, the Internet always offered something new. His work circumstances allowed him free, instant access to the Internet as well as a laptop computer to use on the road. Before long Alan found himself taking breaks at work with his office door closed while visiting his favorite, member-only, online porn sites. Despite regularly coming to work at six or seven in the morning to catch the stock market, Alan would often stay after closing time, taking advantage of the quiet and the freedom from his wife to download pornography and masturbate in his office. As he had seven successful years with this company, no one paid much attention to his schedule or day-to-day activities.

Several times while in the office, Alan met women in online chat rooms, exchanged photos with them, and had "virtual sex"—that is, masturbating while chatting. However, this experience wasn't totally satisfying; he wanted to be able to see and touch these women. Though he had never had sex with another woman outside of his marriage, Alan began flirting with the idea of meeting some of these women in a local hotel or when out of town on business.

Alan had read the human resources memo stating, "Use of the Internet for purposes other than directly work related is strictly prohibited." But he wrote it off because he spent so much legitimate company time on the Internet anyway. He determined that it was nobody's business where he went on the Internet.

One afternoon, while Alan was out of the office, a routine computer upgrade revealed the enormous amount of pornographic material in his work computer. Thoroughly embarrassed and frightened, he promised himself and his supervisor that he would never again use the computer at work for sexual purposes. He told his boss it was a "new fascination" and "something that all the guys sometimes do." He was given a written warning.

Three weeks later, while masturbating at his office computer after hours, Alan was unexpectedly interrupted by a cleaning person. Shocked by what she saw, she reported it to her supervisor, who in turn reported it to human resources. The next day when he returned to work, Alan was immediately fired by his supervisor. When later reviewing the contents of his laptop and office computer, the company found more than 2,500 sexual images saved in Alan's computer files and links to 185 porn sites maintained in his "Favorite Places to Visit" folder.

Alan's story provides many insights into the unmanageable circumstances involved in a life given over to cyber pornography and sexual chat. Neither a casual occurrence nor an idle play experience, Alan's behavior clearly reflects a pattern of escalating use combined with denial of obvious potential consequences.

THE POWER OF DENIAL

Like Alan, others with an addiction will continually carry out patterns of behaviors or activities despite negative consequences to themselves or others. It is almost as if addicts refuse to see or don't understand that their behavior is causing them and others pain or loss. Unlike healthier people who notice when a particular experience or situation is causing problems, people caught up in addictions ignore or deny the seriousness of their actions so they can continue doing them. This process of minimizing consequences, avoiding responsibility for their actions, and rationalizing obviously problematic behaviors is called *denial*. Those addicted to cybersex have a great deal of denial.

Denial subtly insinuates itself into the mind of addicts, encouraging them and increasingly insulating them from reality. Those obsessed with cybersex don't originally intend to ruin their marriage, abandon their career, or get arrested. Yet, often, they end up in these very circumstances, arriving there by incrementally becoming more involved with the intensity and arousal of online sex. As the behaviors and time spent online increase, they become less able to see how their mounting real-life problems are connected to their virtual online sex life. Compulsive cybersex users cannot hear and will not listen to the complaints, concerns, or criticisms of those around them who see what is happening and are willing to say something about it. Nor will they respond to their increasingly neglected career, family life, or even lack of sleep! Cybersex addicts will write off or dismiss these clear warning signs by accusing others of nagging or asking too much of them. Even worse, they will blame the very same troubled family, problematic job, or loneliness for their irritability and exhaustion. They use their career to justify online (escape/relaxation) time—and the resulting distraction and fatigue further escalate the problem.

TYPES OF DENIAL

As noted in chapter 2, the arousal and intensity of the sexual experience, combined with the hidden and compulsive nature of an addictive disorder, create an extraordinarily powerful, druglike state in which someone addicted to cybersex increasingly indulges. To obtain unlimited access to the resources (computer, time alone, Internet), cybersex addicts must find ways to explain—both to themselves and loved ones—why they are so involved with the computer and so unavailable elsewhere. This process of denial escalates the problem, making it more difficult for users and those around them to ascertain what is actually going wrong. Denial takes many forms. A few examples of denial by cybersex addicts in recovery follow.

Entitlement

I just said to myself, Look how hard I am working. I am giving to the family and the company, working nights and some weekends too. There really is no time left for me. There is no time when I can just do what I want to do without interruption or obligation to others. I deserve a little pleasure in life too! If I spend a few hours here and there online, getting off on a little fantasy, it is my only reward for all the work that I do and all that I give to others.

> —*Jeff, a forty-one-year-old married executive with two children, fired after three written warnings not to look at Internet porn sites at work*

Blame

It was never my fault. I just thought, Who wouldn't be checking out women online with the lousy sex life I have at home? Ever since the babies were born, we never have time, and she has put on so much weight. Even when we were having sex, it wasn't anywhere as exciting or interesting as the online chats and conversations I get into. Some of these women are really wild and I get to explore some things I feel like I can't even talk about at home.

> —*Frank, a forty-two-year-old man heavily*
> *into nightly transsexual and bondage*
> *membership services and chats*

Minimization

I figured I was no different. So many of my friends are involved in this Internet thing too. They go online, meet guys for dates, have sex, and then brag about it the next day. My behavior is similar to what I read about in the newspaper or watch on the TV news. Besides, I have been single a long time. While I wait for a relationship, I might as well get all I can. I am not in danger; I can handle myself. Anyone I meet online at least has the money for a computer and the knowledge to use one, so I'm not going to meet any maniacs, right? Besides, I can tell when someone is too weird or into drugs from the kinds of things they write me.

> —*Sam, a thirty-one-year-old man, "found himself"*
> *going to strangers' houses to have sex four to five*
> *nights a week after meeting them online*

Justification

I kept telling myself, "This is what single men do. If I'm not in a relationship, then I need some kind of sexual excitement. It's not like going to the adult bookstores or collecting porn videos. I spend less money on this than on the lousy dating relationships I have been in the last year anyway. Besides, it's a whole lot better than sitting around and watching TV all night. When I come home after work, I can find excitement and distraction without ever having to leave my apartment. You can't beat that."

> —Dave, a twenty-three-year-old single mechanic
> who was spending three to five hours nightly
> watching, trading, and downloading online porn
> from membership Web sites and chat rooms

Rationalization

This is how I looked at it: I'm not having affairs like other women I know, and I am not even flirting with the doctors at work, though I know some other nurses who do. If I get online to have my secret little intrigues, no one really gets hurt and nothing becomes of it. Lots of women read romance novels or watch soap operas, and they aren't doing anything wrong, so why am I?

> —Suzanne, a thirty-six-year-old nurse who,
> after chatting online with a stranger for four months,
> left her marriage of seven years to be with this man;
> her husband never even knew that she went online

CONSEQUENCES OF CYBERSEX ADDICTION

People often first seek help when their sexual behaviors create serious problems in other areas of their lives. Only problems severe enough to get the cybersex addicts' attention or that of others around them can break through the strong insulation of denial described above. Emotional problems, neglect of health and self-care, relationship blowups, sexual problems, career difficulties, family dysfunction, and legal and financial difficulties can all result from the person's substitution of cybersex for real life.

Emotional

Emotionally, I felt guilt and shame that led to isolation and loneliness. This was a part of my life I could not (did not want to) share with my wife. It drove a wedge between us. I was depressed at times because I felt trapped and unable to break free from this obsession. It was scary.

—A forty-five-year-old married man

While many hours at a time were wasted in this endeavor, it never seemed to really satisfy me. Oh, it would for the moment or while I was actually viewing the files, but the letdown and guilt afterward were a real downer. I found myself risking everything—wife, family, reputation—in pursuit of this compulsion. It was when I began to view it as a compulsion that I knew I had a serious problem. But I did not and could not stop. It was only when my wife found some Web-temp [pornographic] files on our home computer that I was forced to finally confront the problem.

—A forty-seven-year-old married man

Cybersex use consumed my life. I was to the point where just closing my eyes would bring on an uncontrollable need to feed my addictive fantasies. The pictures viewed would haunt me day and night. I couldn't look at another person without some filthy thought coming into my mind.

—A thirty-five-year-old married woman

Those obsessed with cybersex face the emotional challenge of living a double life. Keeping secrets, telling lies, minimizing and altering situations and circumstances to cover up realities, lying to self—these are the realities of addiction. Cybersex addicts feels as if they are living two lives, one that takes place in a virtual reality online and another lived in the real world. The online life is one of fantasy, arousal, and distraction. Endless possibilities abound for intrigue, flirtation, and sexual distraction. Time does not really exist on the Net, nor do day-to-day responsibilities, similar to a Las Vegas casino. The online world is a never-ending ride with something or someone new always waiting, just a mouse click away.

Absorption in so much distraction, arousal, and fantasy, while continuing to manage the responsibilities, disappointments, and challenges of the real world creates a gap that widens each day the user acts out his or her obsession with cybersex. As the sexual acting out continues, the cybersex user becomes increasingly irritable, controlling, withdrawn, and exhausted. By the time help is sought, many are in fully expressed anxious and depressive states, driven by ongoing fears of being found out, underlying shame, despair, and for some, self-hatred. Initially, many cybersex users engage in online sexual activity seeking excitement and distraction from their problems. Unfortunately, cybersex activity often creates more serious problems than it resolves.

Self-Care

As their behaviors progress, cybersex addicts have little time for good self-care and physical maintenance. Health suffers as they get increasingly less sleep. Being online long after others have gone to bed or rising in the middle of the night to access the Internet, cybersex addicts lose their sense of healthy boundaries. "Just a few more minutes" turns into hours as the addict searches for the next perfect body or person with whom to chat or masturbate over. In order to avoid confrontations from a concerned spouse or being caught in the act with a sexual or romantic partner online, they give up precious sleep time for the sexual activity.

Besides sleep, other aspects of physical health may suffer.

The Internet chat environment creates an atmosphere of immediacy and intensity in which concerns about safety and self-care are forgotten. Often, resolution of this intense arousal state can be satisfied only by offline (real-life) encounters with casual partners, some of whom may be dangerous people or may be infected with sexually transmitted diseases. Here is Aaron's story:

> I shudder when I recall the risks I took during my active sex addiction. More than once, arriving at a stranger's home at midnight after chatting online for more than two hours, I'd be excited and filled with anticipation. With no condom available, I'd put aside my "usual cautions" of safe sex and have unprotected oral and anal sex; health considerations did not even enter my mind. However, as I walked out of the stranger's home, I was immediately filled with fear and self-loathing, wondering if I'd have to pay a terrible price for this impulsive sexual encounter. I never had much time to think about my HIV risk, however; I had to focus on the more immediate problem of explaining my 2 A.M. arrival to my partner, who was waiting at home.

Although people can't get a sexually transmitted disease from having online sex, 40 percent of cybersex addicts in one survey eventually progressed to real-life sexual encounters, often including unsafe sex.[1]

Relationships, Intimacy, and Sexuality

> It created a wall between us. I avoided intimate conversation so I wouldn't have to answer questions from her that would reveal those secretive and shameful events. As for our sexual relationship, increased sex with myself resulted in less sex with my wife. An increasing preoccupation with body parts

on the screen transferred into a preoccupation with body parts
of real people.

—A sixty-four-year-old married man

Online relationships (often rationalized as "not really an affair") and sexual and romantic real-life encounters with
strangers met online can produce tremendously destructive
consequences for those in a committed relationship. Obsession
with cyberporn, online images, video exchange, or other isolating masturbatory activity leaves primary relationships flat
and drained of meaning. Spouses and significant others, often
confused by the emotional and physical distancing of the addict, may blame themselves for their relationship problems
and judge themselves inadequate. Sexuality, affection, honesty,
and bonding all suffer, as cybersex addicts become increasingly fixated on their solo and anonymous sexual experiences.
For many cybersex addicts who take the leap from virtual reality to actual reality, what was once a "playful distraction"
turns into *very real* affairs.

It affected our sexual relationship greatly. My sexual energy
was saved for the Internet. I lost interest in sex with my partner because I knew there was an unlimited amount of
pictures on the Internet that could "get me off" anytime I preferred. My wife sensed the distance between us. Previously,
it was being connected with each other that formed the base
for our intimate relationship, and this in turn led to sexual
activity. Because we weren't connected, we rarely had sex.
When we did, it was more of an activity than an intimate connection.

—A forty-five-year-old married man

My husband could no longer satisfy me. I wanted what I saw
in the videos and pictures, and was too embarrassed to ask
him for it.

> —*A thirty-five-year-old married woman*

Relationships suffer tragic consequences when cyber-
affairs turn into offline "real" sexual affairs or encounters.
Those discovered to be sexually acting out on the Internet
often must deal with a partner's sense of betrayal, loss of self-
esteem, anger, depression, distancing, and even ending of the
relationship.

In chapter 5, "The Cybersex Widow(er)," we will explore in
greater detail how compulsive cybersex affects those in a committed relationship.

Family Life

In homes where cybersex is routine for one of the spouses,
family life suffers. Basic responsibilities of child care and involvement in family activities become secondary to the cybersex and its resulting emotional distractions and physical
exhaustion. Now having dealt with his problem, William reflects on his experience:

Looking back, I can see that as my cybersex life became more
important, I was spending less and less time playing with the
children after school and on weekends. Today I can't believe I
didn't realize this sooner, because I had been such an active
dad before all this started. After work, instead of joining the
family, I would hole up in the den on the computer until late in
the evening, sometimes skipping dinner altogether. I just
gradually got less involved in figuring out the usual household dilemmas, the child care balancing act, or even helping

with the kids' homework. In retrospect I can see how my wife picked up the slack, taking on more of my responsibilities. When she would challenge me on this, I would just lie and defend myself, saying stuff like, "You don't seem to understand how important it is for me to get this work done," or "Why can't you do your part and keep things out of my way so that I can work in here?" Sometimes I think I even picked fights to justify going in my study and shutting the door on her. It makes me feel really shameful when I think about it.

Sue tells me now that sometimes she was concerned about even leaving the kids with me when she went out to run errands. I would get so involved with whatever I was doing on the computer that she worried I wasn't really watching them and wouldn't hear if they needed me. And forget about any closeness between Sue and me! Making any kind of time for the two of us wasn't even on my radar. My denial about the whole thing only broke down when she finally confronted me and threatened to move out with the kids unless things changed. At that point I just got honest about what I had really been doing online and begged her to forgive me. When she insisted on my going to counseling, I finally agreed that there was a problem.

Compulsive use of the Internet affects all aspects of parenting. In the previous story, William's attention was elsewhere. Read on to see how a cybersex user's inattention to his children may cost him his marriage:

Although my wife tried for years to get pregnant, I realize that my involvement with our daughter was meager at best. The cybersex use started while we were pregnant with Jessica and just got worse after she was born. I think I really missed out on the special things like her first steps and words. I would spend hours on the computer at night, insisting that it was not interfering with our family time. Many days I spent catching up on sleep, missing out on time with our child.

The event that caused our separation was when I actually neglected Jessica one day while I was in the bedroom having cybersex. Jessica was down for a nap, and I was supposed to listen to the baby monitor while my wife went to work. Somehow I left the monitor in another room, thinking I would just turn on the computer for a few minutes. Before I knew it, several hours had passed. My wife came home to find me masturbating in front of the computer and our daughter screaming her head off. My wife left me the next day.

Now that we are separated, I actually spend more time with Jessica than I did before, because when I go to see her, I am really being with her, not just passing time to get back to the computer.

—*Frank, a twenty-eight-year-old man,*
separated after an eight-year marriage

In other cases, the children are directly exposed to pornography:

I know the boys have gotten into my "Special Photos" file on the PC. They've walked in when I was chatting and saw the sexual chat rooms where I spend time. They've even told me to take those pictures off the computer, that "it's gross." I told them it was none of their business, but I think they've lost respect for me. Now I try to be more discreet about it with the kids, but I'm sure they've heard my wife and me arguing about it.

—*Armand, a forty-two-year-old man,*
married seventeen years

Even if the children are not exposed to online pornography or do not know how their parents are spending their time, they may be harmed because of their parent's emotional withdrawal, causing tension and arguments in the home. Denial may, at first, prevent the cybersex user from seeing the family consequences.

Careers

Searching for online pornography and sexual encounters in the workplace is dangerous business. Most larger companies now have policies regarding such behavior. Human resource policies usually include a verbal and/or written warning for the first offense, followed by immediate dismissal for a recurrence. In denial of the potential consequences, cybersex addicts will often excuse the behavior by telling themselves, "They won't find out it was me" or "This is no big deal, I look online only after hours, not on company time" or "Lots of employees do this. I have seen pictures on other people's computers a million times." Denial will kick in. They will ignore or try to get around memos and warnings, finding the behavior too enticing and accessible to stop.

In the past, tolerant businesses looked the other way at such behavior. Now, corporations large and small are actively seeking to stop cybersex viewing and romantic chat in the work environment. The law now permits an employer to review and read an employee's e-mail and to subject the e-mail's author to scrutiny and reproach. Computers networked into a mainframe or using a central ISDN line often have filters and programs designed to monitor the online activities of workers. Personal computers and laptops are routinely checked when in maintenance or while having software upgrades. Employees unable or unwilling to change their behaviors are now routinely being fired:

> I lost my job and could not find anything I wanted to do, so I spent all day on the computer while my wife worked two jobs

to try to keep up financially. In the last couple of years before we split up, I ran up about $29,000 on our credit cards due to my cybersex activities. My addiction cost me my marriage.

—A thirty-eight-year-old man, now divorced

He put both his job and mine in jeopardy. He did this by using my government computer account and surfing on the Internet at his work during work hours. He had more than one hundred computer disks filled with alphabetized porn images in his work computer.

—A forty-four-year-old woman, now separated

Finances

One of the great benefits of the Internet is the low cost at which an endless amount of information and enjoyment can be accessed. However, it also provides enormous opportunities for people to benefit financially; for example, anyone who wishes to make money online can charge for access to their Web sites. In the sexual arena, even though there is a great deal of free material available, Web sites run by "professionals" provide more consistency and greater depth of content on specific types of pornography. Some of these, called *membership sites*, require the viewer to pay a monthly membership access fee. Other sites charge for the amount of time the user spends viewing materials and images.

The intensely arousing nature of the sexual content encourages the viewer to keep looking and searching for more. This type of online experience can become highly expensive for the viewer and lucrative for the operators. It is not unusual for a site to charge several dollars per minute. In one sitting, a viewer can easily spend hundreds of dollars. Specialty sexual services such as live video feeds, live viewing of models, and sexual chats with models cost considerably more per minute, in addition to the initial membership fee. Cybersex addicts who feel ashamed or angry at themselves for the time spent online will often cancel their memberships or even online access. Within a few days, they sign back on and start all over again. All of this can be very expensive. One man reported having racked up more than $8,000 on his credit card in a two-month period, and he could not stop.

In addition to the direct costs of cybersex activities, compulsive use can demand large sums of money for upgrades to computer equipment. If the online activities progress to telephone contact and offline encounters, the expenses mount quickly:

> Even though I did not purchase anything online, I spent thousands of dollars on my addiction. I pushed to purchase a computer and wanted extra graphics capabilities (for the pictures on my games, I told my wife), and the new equipment that made downloading pictures faster. My wife wanted to wait until this new technology went down in price (which it did), but I insisted until she finally gave in.
>
> —*A twenty-nine-year-old man, married four years*

> I spent money in traveling, buying gifts, purchasing phone cards, staying in motels, and buying lovers dinner, outlays which have drained our mutual finances. This has created financial stress for both of us and made her increasingly want independence from our "marriage."
>
> —*A forty-four-year-old lesbian, speaking of a four-year relationship*

Legal

Access to illegal sexual activities and content is readily available through the Internet. This includes the illegal exchange of images of child pornography, graphic sexual violence, mutilation, bestiality, and sexual death or "snuff photos." Unknown to the average online viewer, however, many of the sites through which these images are accessed are either monitored by or managed by various governmental watchdog agencies. Larger online service companies such as America Online (AOL), Earthlink, and Sprint are required to report to the government any activity that might involve any of the above materials. Stories like the following account are occurring with increasing frequency around the country.

> Kevin had always felt aroused by looking at and being around young teens. For many years, girls aged eleven to fourteen had been a strong part of his sexual fantasy life. Throughout his twenties, while dating and enjoying sex with women his own age, Kevin recalled having "crushes" on much younger girls who were friends of his little sister. Though never actually acting upon these thoughts, he would use them as subjects for masturbation and sexual fantasy. Now in his early thirties, married, with toddlers of his own, Kevin had pushed these "Lolita" interests to the back of his psyche and was enjoying married life and a pleasant sexual life.
>
> The pregnancy and birth of his third child was hard on the whole family. Kevin's wife was uncomfortable and exhausted, and was forced to rest much of the time. Kevin had to take on the responsibilities of raising two small children and most of the financial burden as well. It wasn't long before the pressures of his family life, challenges at work, and the long hours of caring for his wife began to weigh on him. Initially on impulse, Kevin turned to the computer in the late evenings after the kids were in bed and his wife sound asleep. Impressed at first by the variety of content on the Internet, he would spend hours exploring various interests and hobbies. Later, when he discovered the ready availability of explicit sexual material, the

impulse became a habit. Within months, Kevin was online until late at night, sometimes into the early hours of the morning.

It wasn't long before Kevin discovered "teen photo galleries" and "young teen chats." At that point, his long-suppressed fantasy life became increasingly more real, as Kevin was for the first time exposed to actual images and stories about underage girls. Lulled by the safety of his home computer, Kevin didn't even consider the illegality of his actions as he transported and explored child pornography over the Internet. Before long he was regularly downloading and masturbating to photos of young teenage girls and going to chat rooms to exchange pornographic images with others.

What Kevin did not know is that several of the teen sites he visited were under regular observation by the FBI, which is one of the agencies that closely monitor Internet use, particularly the illegal exchange of child pornography. The inevitable knock at his door, seizure of his computer hard drive, and subsequent arrest came as a total shock to Kevin and his family. The evidence, when uncovered, included hundreds of legal pornographic images in the computer along with dozens of illegal photos of young teens in various states of compromise and exploitation. Kevin was prosecuted and charged as a sex offender for engaging in the traffic of child pornography across state lines.

CONCLUSIONS

The average person who begins viewing online pornography and engaging in sexually oriented Internet activities often does so as recreation, taking it no further than occasional use and stopping when the activity appears to interfere or cause problems in life and in relationships. For some, however, the activities become compulsive, and stopping becomes increasingly more difficult. This eventually creates serious consequences for the viewer. In the 1999 Cooper survey of more than Internet users, 8.3 percent had online behavior patterns severe enough to be considered sexually compulsive.[2] The Cybersex Addiction Checklist in appendix 1 (pages 196–197) provides a good summary of the behavior that constitutes cybersex addiction.

For the vulnerable man or woman, the intensity of the Internet is comparable to that of crack cocaine for the budding drug addict. In both cases, the addiction progresses rapidly, and so do the negative consequences. Using the voices of actual men and women who have become ensnared in the cybersex web, this chapter has outlined some of these consequences, which can include emotional, relationship, family, career, financial, and legal disasters.

So far, our discussion has focused primarily on overtly sexual Internet activities, such as viewing pornography and engaging in real-time online sex. Although both genders are involved in these activities, men more than women are aroused by visual images. Typically, women pursue the lure of romance on the Internet, not pornographic images. Romance on the Internet can be highly addictive for some users, luring them into the unrealistic promise of an ideal relationship. People may fly halfway across the country to meet an online "soul mate" while breaking up long-term relationships. The phenomenon of cybersex romance will be explored in the next chapter.

FOUR

Fantasy and Romance Addiction on the Internet

◉ ◉ ◉

Annette, a thirty-seven-year-old divorced nurse, was searching online for a long-term relationship:

> When I met Kevin online, I was sure I'd finally found my soul mate. We worked in related fields and were both interested in the same things. It was so easy to "chat" with him—in a short time I felt I'd known him forever. Since I live in California and he lives in Delaware, it was several months before we actually met. We exchanged daily e-mails, sent each other our photographs, and talked on the phone a few times. Our messages did eventually contain some sexual innuendos, but nothing explicit. Finally, we agreed to meet for a weekend in Chicago. By then I believed I was in love with him.
>
> We arranged to rendezvous at O'Hare Airport on a Friday evening and went out to dinner. Kevin was as good-looking as his picture, and I could tell he was pleased with what he saw as well. But as the meal progressed, I began to suspect that I had made a big mistake with this guy. Throughout dinner Kevin was controlling, overbearing, and consistently interrupting my comments. He insisted on ordering dinner for me without my feedback and talked endlessly about his plans for

our next meeting without even asking my opinion. While chain-smoking and consuming nonstop martinis, he waxed on about how I really was "the girl of his dreams" and that he "couldn't wait" until I moved closer to be with him. I began to feel increasingly more uncomfortable with the intensity of his approach, especially considering we had never really met before!

I started fantasizing about getting back to the airport to catch a late-night flight home. Unfortunately, my plane ticket was nonrefundable, so I felt obligated to stick with it and spend the weekend in Chicago. Thankfully, I had suggested we stay in separate hotel rooms while we got to know each other and was glad to retreat to my own room at the end of the first evening—that is, until his first knock at the door at 1 A.M. I was tired and apprehensive, but let him in anyway, as he appeared upset. He sat down and began talking about his last few relationships and how unhappy he had been. He hoped that this time it would work out and I would be "the one." It was clear to me that he had continued drinking after our dinner together and was now quite drunk. He began to make sexual suggestions and asked if we could lie together and cuddle. As he became more insistent, I started to feel truly frightened for my safety and asked him to leave. It was only when I threatened to call security that he agreed to go back to his own room. Early the next morning, on the first plane I could get home (by this time airfare was no object), I tried to figure out how I could have so misjudged his character and gotten myself into this situation in the first place.

Annette's experience illustrates the most salient characteristics of Internet romance: Love connections are easy to make, but the nature of Internet communication encourages fantasy while ignoring reality. For single people who are just looking for a good time, the only loss when reality intrudes may be some hours wasted at the computer and some money spent on phone calls or real-life meetings. But when emotions become all-consuming and romance and sex become the focus of the online connection, the stakes are higher and the consequences potentially devastating. When online users are married or in committed relationships with real-life partners, whole families can be torn apart by seemingly innocuous online romances.

This chapter explores the nature of romantic love, how the computer fosters and perpetuates fantasy, and how those who are addicted to romance or sex are likely candidates to get caught in the Net. It also discusses the pitfalls to avoid when dating on the Internet. The tendency of online communication to foster fantasy makes it particularly appealing to "romance addicts." Although traditionally a role taken by women, both sexes can be found among romance addicts. On the Internet, women sex addicts are more likely to be seeking romance, in contrast to male sex addicts who are more likely to spend their time viewing pornographic images.

MEETING ONLINE: THE MEDIUM IS THE MESSAGE

In our culture, many people are isolated by circumstance, lack of community, and the time constraints of work. Even urban dwellers surrounded by masses of people seem to have fewer and fewer opportunities to meet potential romantic partners. Without a doubt, the Internet has become a major resource for meeting new people. Online dating services and personals are a rapidly burgeoning feature of the Internet. People typically meet each other by participating in a chat room or discussion group devoted to some particular interest.

Meeting others on the Internet does have its advantages. The Internet can quickly and inexpensively link people who may be hundreds or thousands of miles apart, thereby facilitating communication. The current use of writing as the primary form of communication on the Internet is also beneficial when meeting new people. In contrast to live encounters, first impressions on the Internet are based on what is said, not on one's physical appearance. Given the huge emphasis in our culture on looks, it can be an enormous advantage for a less physically attractive person to be able to engage in an extended dialogue with a potential romantic partner before meeting face-to-face. Another advantage is that people have plenty of time to express themselves as fully and as positively as possible. In live interactions, shy people may have so much anxiety about how to respond to new acquaintances that they barely pay attention to the spoken words. The Internet, by contrast, offers more time to digest what is said and to formulate an articulate, thoughtful, and relevant reply. For people who do not excel at verbal communication, especially when first dating, the Internet provides an opportunity to be presented in the most positive light. This is particularly true for e-mail, which can be sent and downloaded at one's convenience. But even in "real-time" chat rooms, messages can be revised and reviewed before being transmitted.

Here are some other advantages of Internet introductions:

- Whereas newspaper ads limit people to describing themselves in twenty or thirty words, computer matching "profiles" allow a description of several hundred words in many different areas. This detailed and extensive information helps potential partners decide whether they are truly interested in the other person.

- The cost of computer matching is a small fraction of off-line matchmaking services.
- For nonurban dwellers, the pool of potential Internet matches is much larger online than in a local community, if one is willing to travel.
- Participation in topic-focused chat rooms and e-mail lists introduces participants to many other people with similar interests.

Because of the Internet's apparent anonymity, many people feel less inhibited communicating via e-mail than in person. As a result, they are willing to express their feelings more openly and honestly. A willingness to share emotions and reveal personal vulnerability can lead to a sense of intimacy much more rapidly over the Internet than in an offline relationship.

Virtual Love: An Object Lesson

Internet dating, with its built-in barriers to full knowledge of the other person, is the perfect setup for "falling in love." Sometimes the outcome of online fantasy romances is good; many people have heard stories of couples who met online and are living "happily ever after." Unfortunately, for every success story there is at least one of unhappiness or even danger. Stories range from failed expectations to disrupted marriages and even violence.

A poignant tale of reality's inability to live up to fantasy was told by Meghan Daum in her first-person account "Virtual Love."[1] Daum wrote of her online relationship with Pete: "I was a desired person, the object of a blind man's gaze. . . . He told me that he thought about me all the time, though we both knew that the 'me' in his mind consisted largely of himself." She became equally obsessed with him.

When, after several months of e-mails, Pete flew from

California to New York to meet Meghan, it was a disaster: "He talked so much that I wanted to cry. . . . It was all wrong. The physical world had invaded our space. I wanted Pete out of my apartment. . . . I berated myself for not liking him, for wanting to like him more than I had wanted anything in such a long time. I was horrified by the realization that I had invested so heavily in a made-up character. . . . If Pete and I had met at a party, we probably wouldn't have spoken to each other for more than ten minutes." Their months-long intense fantasy romance died as a result of a single real-life meeting.

Computer Dating Caveats

What went wrong with Meghan and Pete's "relationship"? One possible explanation is that the medium of the Internet contains elements of omission (missing cues) and commission (ease of deception) that encourage creating fantasies of the other person. For example:

- *Computer communication lacks many cues,* such as facial and vocal expression and body language. These missing cues are inevitably filled in with completely inaccurate fantasy images of the other person, even when he or she is not deliberately deceptive.
- *On the computer, most people intentionally lie* about some aspect of themselves. Personal photographs sent to others or put on matchmaking profiles are often out of date and sometimes are of another person: When one man finally went to meet an attractive woman with whom he'd been e-mailing through an online matchmaking service, he told of showing up at her door and being introduced to her daughter, whom he recognized as the person whose picture was on his date's computer profile!

- *The very nature of computer interaction significantly alters the way communication takes place.* For one, e-mail correspondence forces each person to take turns. As a result, the person who constantly interrupts and dominates a live discussion would go undetected. Moreover, because e-mail correspondence allows each person time to formulate his or her thoughts and express them optimally, it can disguise when the person at the other end is socially awkward or too shy to carry on a face-to-face conversation. Marshall McLuhan, famed mid-twentieth-century analyst of the effects of media on our culture, recognized that in large part "the media is the message." This concept is especially true of the Internet. By the very nature of Internet communication, which is sequential, the opportunity to interrupt is eliminated. Particularly with e-mail correspondence, but even in chat rooms, people can complete their thoughts without the fear of being stopped midstream. In this respect, the Internet forces people to be polite.
- *The relative anonymity of the computer can foster "pseudo-intimacy,"* making people more willing to reveal themselves in ways they would not normally do in a real-life meeting. The perceived sense of trust and acceptance leads to the illusion that they know each other very well, whereas this is often false.
- *People engaged in online relationships tend to spend more and more time online rather than developing relationships in the real world.* This may lead them to become increasingly dependent on the online relationship to meet their needs, thereby reducing their practice of socializing in the real world. This developing dependency, plus the perceived anonymity and safety of the computer, encourages the sexualization of online relationships.

- *Correspondence that begins as an innocent friendship has the potential to turn into erotic dialogue and then into full-blown cybersex.* This may be augmented by the use of cameras and the telephone. The fantasy and illusion inherent in such relationships often leads to unrealistic expectations of what a face-to-face encounter with the same person might be like.

As so many of the stories in this book emphasize, even without overt sexualization, the power and intensity of fantasy relationships can become so great that people married or in committed relationships have left their jobs and families, burned bridges, and traveled long distances to be with someone they've never met, but with whom they're convinced they're in love. Occasionally, these relationships do work out, but all too often they are disastrous. In many cases, as with Meghan Daum's experience above, a real-life meeting reveals the chasm between fantasy and reality, often leading to a quick ending of the relationship. When cybersex leads to an offline affair, some people may be fortunate enough to have a forgiving partner who is willing to take them back. The not-so-lucky others may lose their family, home, and job. Ina, a thirty-eight-year-old professional woman who'd been married seventeen years, nearly lost her marriage as a result of a long-distance online relationship that she claims was neither sexual nor romantic. It did, nonetheless, become all-consuming and compulsive:

The Power of Fantasy: Ina's Story

It started with a series of e-mails with a man I had never met before but had reason to be in contact with through my work. Elliot is an eloquent writer, as I am; he and I found amusement in that. It escalated. Soon we began to instant message (IM) each other. [IM is an Internet service that allows back-and-forth chatting between people, much like a telephone conversation, only in print.] In this way we became constantly available to each other online throughout the workday. We arranged to coordinate our hours. When he went to his office earlier, I woke up earlier. When he stayed at work later, I stayed online later. Then it became weekends too. While much of our conversation was professional, it became more personal in nature.

His marriage was grim; mine was too. I viewed our online relationship as a game. We even discussed the infidelity issue. We both justified our continued dialogue. Although there was no discussion of love or romance, or getting together in any permanent way, our contacts progressed and escalated in content and intensity—I was consumed by his e-mails, IM, and phone calls. I was behaving compulsively, and I was not able to control it. Eventually I stopped getting anything done of my own work. I became progressively more isolated and withdrawn. I stopped being with my kids unless I had to. I was short-tempered and distant from them, and they reacted by misbehaving. It was very stressful on the entire family. It also negatively impacted my sexual relationship with my husband.

Eventually, I had the opportunity to travel on business to St. Louis, where Elliot lived, and we arranged to meet. I immediately became preoccupied with fantasies about the meeting. The anticipation was very stirring. Although I encouraged my husband, Ben, to stay at home, in the end he came along anyway. Nonetheless, Elliot and I managed to meet. The meeting was a rude awakening; Elliot was nothing like what I had imagined. His humor, his ability to paint wonderful word pictures, his sensitivity—somehow all those qualities I'd liked so much about him were restricted to his writing. On the computer he had unlimited time to polish his communications. In person, he was inarticulate while at the same time self-righteous and critical. Mark my words: The fantasy is much better!

While we were in St. Louis, Ben became suspicious and I disclosed my online relationship with Elliot to him. He just about lost it! He thought I was going to run off with this guy. He asked me if I wanted a divorce. Despite my many reassurances to the contrary, he remained very upset. On the way home, he decided to even the score by disclosing to me an old affair he'd had. He was obviously trying to hurt me and was being very cruel. We are now in counseling, dealing with the fundamental relationship issues of secrecy, lying, mistrust, and infidelity.

Ina's story shows how even in the absence of overt romance or sex on the Internet, a woman's search for a fantasy connection can be destructive to both herself and her family. In therapy, Ina continues to sort out how she was drawn so powerfully and compulsively into her online relationship. After all, she didn't have a history of any Internet romances.

Fantasy versus Reality

Here are some warning signs that you've developed a fantasy relationship on the Internet:

- receiving an online friend's latest e-mail is the highlight of your day
- you spend work hours obsessing about the person
- you give up time normally spent with friends to stay at home chatting online
- you think you're in love even though you've never met

An offline meeting may completely alter your feelings about that person. People already married or in committed relationships who find themselves in the above scenario might consider counseling.

Without the reality check that real-life meetings provide, it is hard not to attribute to a new online friend all those wonderful qualities being sought in an ideal life partner. This tendency is enhanced by the pseudo-intimacy of Internet communication, which can foster soulful sharing of feelings while ignoring the realities of the person's life. Such attribution is normal; under the same circumstances we are all likely to do it. The Internet is the ideal medium for fantasy romances. To make this clear, consider the characteristics of romantic love.

ROMANTIC LOVE

In his book *We: Understanding the Psychology of Romantic Love*, Robert A. Johnson wrote the following:

> Romantic love doesn't just mean loving someone; it means being "in love." When we are "in love," we believe we have found the ultimate meaning of life, revealed in another human being. We feel we are finally completed, that we have found the missing parts of ourselves. Life suddenly seems to have a wholeness, a superhuman intensity that lifts us high above the ordinary plane of existence.[2]

No wonder romantic love is so powerful and so sought after! Unfortunately, the circumstances favoring romantic love also ensure that it does not last forever. Romantic love flourishes when people don't know each other well; when they are unsure of the other's caring and commitment; when there are barriers to their encounters, such as physical distance between them or the need for secrecy; and when there are limits on the time they spend together. This lack of real knowledge about the other person guarantees that each will only see the person's desirable characteristics based on fantasy rather than reality.

When they get to know each other better, disillusionment is inevitable; the couple then has the opportunity to work on the tasks of developing real intimacy. These tasks are most clearly described by Bader and Pearson in their book *In Quest of the Mythical Mate*.[3] Long-term relationships exhibit a predictable pattern, in which the early stage of romantic love is followed by a stage of distancing or disillusionment. During this period, many marriages and committed relationships falter and end. In successful relationships, this difficult stage is resolved and followed by "rapprochement," a coming back together based on a more realistic appreciation for the other person.

Healthy romantic love encourages playfulness and intimacy, and it can bring a fresh sense of self, learned through being with a new partner. Romance, with or without sex, revitalizes personal growth as each new relationship forces new insights and self-knowledge. The beginning stages of a potential love relationship are often intense and exciting. Most people easily relate to the "rush" of first love and romance, that stuff of songs, greeting cards, and warm memories. Healthy intimacy, however, is characterized by more than romance, intensity, and sex. Intimacy is an experience of knowing a person well over time. Loving, longer-term relationships develop by using those early exhilarating times as ways to build a bridge toward deeper, longer-term closeness.

It can be difficult for anyone to understand how love or sexuality can be exploited or evolve into destructive patterns of addiction and compulsion. Yet, for the romance addict, romantic love, sexuality, and the closeness these relationships offer are experiences often filled with pitfalls, anxiety, and eventual pain. Attempting to love in a sometimes-chaotic emotional world of desperation and despair, fearful of being alone or rejected, but trapped by unconscious fears of being overwhelmed by closeness, romance addicts endlessly long for that "special" relationship with someone who will need them and love them.

Yet this constant search—which involves endless intrigue, flirtations, sexual liaisons, and affairs—often leaves a path of destruction and negative consequences. Without support and direction, romance addicts usually find few options to resolve these painful circumstances other than by engaging in even more searching, an escalating cycle of desperation and loss. Just when seemingly "safe" in the rush of a new romantic affair or liaison, the troubled romance addict often grows steadily more unhappy and fearful and ends up pushing new partners away or starting new relationships before the current one has ended. Constantly running away or chasing those who are emotionally unavailable leaves the romance addict again longing for another new intense "love" experience. Maybe next time, the "right one" will come along.

Unlike psychologically healthy people, who seek partnership and sex to enrich their lives rather than to make them feel whole, romance addicts search for something outside of themselves (a person, relationship, or experience) to provide the emotional and life stability they themselves lack. Often either hopelessly overcommitted, or isolated and deprived of outside support, these people are drawn to find someone "out there" to fill their endless needs. Similar to drug addicts or alcoholics, romance and sex addicts use their arousing romantic/sexual experiences to "fix" themselves and remain emotionally stable. As a result, they make poor partner choices. Compatibility becomes based on "how much you want me," "whether or not you will ever leave me," or "how intense our sex life is" rather than on whether you might truly become a peer, friend, and companion.

Addictive relationships are characterized over time by unhealthy dependency, guilt, and abuse (emotional, physical, or sexual). Convinced of their lack of worth and not feeling truly lovable, romance addicts will use seduction, control, guilt, and manipulation to attract and hold on to romantic partners. At times, despairing of this cycle of unhappy affairs, broken relationships, and sexual liaisons, some romance addicts may have "swearing off" periods (like the bulimic/anorexic cycles of overeaters), believing that "not being in the game" will solve the problem. Those same problems of intimacy and fear reappear when, tired of being alone, the romance addict re-enters the playing field.

Here are the twelve signs of romance addiction:

1. feeling detached or unhappy when in a relationship, yet feeling desperate and alone when out of a relationship
2. avoiding sex or relationships for long periods of time to "solve the problem"
3. being unable to leave unhealthy relationships despite repeated promises to self or others
4. having affairs or intense flirtation and intrigue while already in a relationship
5. returning to previously unmanageable or painful relationships despite promises to self or others
6. repeatedly mistaking sex and romantic intensity for love
7. constantly seeking a sexual partner, new romance, or significant other
8. feeling incapable of or having difficulty in being alone
9. choosing partners who are abusive or emotionally unavailable
10. using sex, seduction, and intrigue to "hook" or hold on to a partner
11. using sex or romantic intensity to tolerate difficult experiences or emotions

12. missing out on important family, career, or social experiences in order to maintain a sexual high or romantic relationship

For the person addicted to fantasy, the above signs or symptoms create a pervasive pattern of emotional instability that inevitably leads to isolation, heartache, and loss. Not everyone who displays any of the above behaviors has an addiction problem. At times, almost everyone experiences skewed judgment upon encountering a difficult person or situation. For romance addicts, however, it becomes the norm, lived over and over again in some form or another. Romance addicts who are not working toward change or recovery do not learn from their consequences and mistakes. It is much easier to blame the partner or lover as being "the problem." It is only when the pain of these behaviors and situations becomes greater than the pain and challenges of creating change that recovery begins.

People who are unable to stop their relentless search for a partner may view most any situation or experience as an opportunity to find that perfect somebody. Upon reflection, many recovering romance addicts report having used some strategy or another all of their lives in an attempt to find and keep sexual and romantic partners. One woman put it this way, "I never once went to a party without wondering who I could get a date with or get into bed with. I always dressed and looked for it." Whether through revealing dress, flirtatious manner, or seductive talk, the romance addict is continually hunting and searching for that special attention, intensity, and arousal that only the latest tryst or liaison can offer. An important part of the recovery process is recognizing those methods used solely to attract and manipulate others. As addicts begin to consciously cast these aside—using the help of support group members, friends, and often therapy—they come to learn their real human worth, lessening the need for superficial, sexualized attention.

CAUGHT ON THE NET WITH A SEX ADDICT

In their efforts to attract and hold on to a man, some women become willing to shortcut the path to intimacy by quickly agreeing to engage in cybersex or phone sex. Often, the outcome is not what the woman had hoped for.

Judy's Story

Consider the story of Judy, a thirty-two-year-old recently divorced woman:

> My husband, Ken, and I met on the Internet six years ago. We didn't actually engage in cybersex, but quickly developed a phone-sex relationship based on dominance and submission. By the time we met in person six months after first meeting online, we were both in love. I agreed to move halfway across the country to be with him. We married a short time later. Unfortunately, real-life sex with him didn't live up to my expectations and was nothing like he promised me on the phone. When he had trouble maintaining an erection, I assumed all the blame, because I was very inexperienced. He was always too tired for real sex with me, and for a long time I didn't know why. I felt lonely and paranoid. He told me to initiate sex more, but then when I did, he'd always turn me down. I felt so confused.
>
> One day I accidentally walked in on Ken while he was sitting at the computer. He was masturbating while typing sexual messages to another woman. It turns out that all along my hus-

band had been having sex with other women through the Internet. Several times I confronted him and threatened to leave. He'd always promise to stop, but he never did. Nonetheless, I would never have left him—I was too terrified to be alone. I was desperate to keep him, especially after our daughter was born.

Recently my husband "fell in love" with another woman on the Internet. Even before he met her in person, he told me he no longer loved me. He left to be with her. This has absolutely devastated me. Until I found out about his cybersex activities, I thought this man was the love of my life—my knight in shining armor—despite our sexual problems. Through therapy and recovery, I'm now discovering our relationship had nothing to do with love—only addiction. It's very depressing to love someone and then have him say, No, it's someone else, and yet we met the same way. If it weren't for our daughter, I think I would have killed myself.

Judy is an example of a woman who, in her quest for romance, unknowingly became involved with a cybersex addict. In her intense desire to please Ken, she willingly had phone sex with him. She assumed that once they developed a real relationship, he would stop the phone sex and settle into a more traditional, monogamous marriage. Not surprisingly, this didn't happen, and Judy continued to "enable" Ken by not following through on her threats to leave. Now, thanks to her therapy, Judy has a clearer understanding of her part in the drama. She wrote:

When Ken was first diagnosed as a sex addict, I assumed it was *his* problem and he needed to "fix" it. I had no idea the role I played in the whole situation. Since he left me, I've begun attending S-Anon [a Twelve Step program for families of sex addicts] and ACOA [Adult Children of Alcoholics] and I see a therapist weekly. I'm reading lots of books on addiction, codependency, and love addiction. I now have a better understanding of my role in getting into this relationship in the first place and am working on improving my self-esteem. I hope that if I get into another relationship, I will make a better choice.

People who are needy, who are looking for another person to make them feel whole, and who have difficulty trusting their own judgment are particularly vulnerable to the lure of a cybersex fantasy romance. After therapy, Judy recognized her own role in jumping into and staying in her dysfunctional relationship. She then took steps to heal herself.

Many women, like Judy, initially go online to meet a compatible dating partner and agree to participate in online sex to expedite the relationship. Some people, in their confusion of sex and love, go online specifically seeking sexual interactions, believing it will somehow win them love. Unfortunately, when two people meet online with the goal of sexual activities, then later attempt to convert the relationship to a more traditional one, there are predictable risks.

MALE ROMANCE ADDICTS

Like many of the women described above, men can also get trapped in the illusory nature of online romance. Although men tend to step deeper into clear-cut porn and overt sexual content than into romantic addiction,[4] there are clearly cases where the rush and excitement of a new online partner can become a potent obsession. These connections may start out as a sexual fix or distraction without the intent for a relationship, but can develop unexpectedly into more. Male sex addicts may engage in multiple online relationships at varying stages. They may be regularly exchanging photos, information, and sexual chat with several people for purely sexual purposes while also engaging romantically online and offline with several others. Like a computer operating system that can keep many "windows" open at one time, the online male sex addict can conduct multiple sexual and romantic engagements simultaneously. Romantic obsession often evolves when the dynamics of an alluring and potentially unavailable partner come into play.

Meeting His Angel: Jeffrey's Story

I nearly lost my wife and kids because of a fantasy. Until recently I could regularly be found in the basement "working on the computer." After the family dinner, I'd spend three to four hours in the basement, several nights a week, intensely involved in online sex. I kept a daily check-in on my favorite sexual chat rooms, seeing who was there, flirting, hitting on women, and exchanging photos. I also subscribed to a service where I could order up "models" who would perform "live sex," in whatever way I requested, while I masturbated. Although I never intended to go further than these activities, I felt myself increasingly drawn to one particular girl named "Angel" who did live online porn. At first I became "involved" with her through watching her perform, and I would specifically request her several times weekly.

Over a three-month period, I spent an unbelievable $3,500 on these computer sessions with Angel. During this time, I increasingly withdrew from my wife and family and found creative ways to lie about where the money was going. Work also became secondary to this cyberaffair, as I was checking in online with her many times throughout the day. I actually became jealous and afraid she would get "involved" with some other guy.

> —*Jeffrey, a married thirty-six-year-old*
> *Web site designer and father of three*

Looking back, Jeff acknowledges that the experience became more intense as he began to pursue the "real girl" rather than the fantasy. The object of his intensity became "getting Angel to want me and to tell me who she really was, to put down her work image and let me in." Jeff's most intense and arousing moments occurred when Angel finally revealed to him her real name and gave him her personal e-mail address. Jeff reports becoming completely hooked at this point after hearing Angel's tragic life story.

After he convinced himself that he might be falling in love with her, he requested a live meeting. In planning this meeting, he made plane and hotel reservations and convincingly lied to his wife and boss about where he was going and why. It was only in the time he spent talking to his children about why "Daddy would be away for a while" that Jeff broke down and realized how out of control he was. At this point, instead of leaving to meet Angel, Jeff went out and sought professional help for his problem.

Like many sex and cybersex addicts, Jeff used the relationship as a power contest: He was trying to get Angel to want him enough to let down her guard and let him in. This became his obsession. The more Angel seemed to count on and need him, alternately pulling away and ignoring him, the more arousing the situation became for him and the more he wanted to see her. These issues of dependency, potential abandonment, power, and obsession frequently become intermingled for the cybersex addict who is active online, seeking to feel important, wanted, and desirable. In the end, this often causes great emotional, personal, and financial losses for the addict and his family.

WOMEN SEX ADDICTS
AND THE COMPUTER

Like chemical dependency, sex addiction affects both men and women. Approximately 25 percent of people in sex addiction recovery programs are women. Just as with alcoholism, admitting sex addiction is more shameful for women than for men. Even our language reflects this difference: A man who has multiple sexual encounters is known as a "skirt chaser," "ladies' man," "stud," or "Don Juan," while a woman who sleeps with many men is called a "slut," "whore," or "nymphomaniac." It is often more difficult for women to own up to their problem and seek help.

As indicated earlier, studies have shown that men are more interested than women in visual sexual activities (viewing pornographic images and films, voyeurism, and so on) and sex with partners who are anonymous or virtual strangers. Women are more likely than men to want romance and relationship as part of their sexual activities.[5] As a result, women are the primary audience for the multimillion-dollar soap opera and romance novel industry. Translated to the Internet, men are more likely than women to download and view pornography. Women prefer chat rooms and personal ads, where they can actually "get to know" men. A preliminary study suggests that women cybersex addicts are more likely than men to seek offline sexual meetings as a result of their online sexual activities.[6] The same woman who identifies with the heroine of a romance novel who is swept off her feet by the man of her dreams now may find herself willing to risk all for the cybersex romance fantasy. Even when having the same goal as a male sex addict—the casual sexual encounter—most female sex addicts lean toward some type of relationship-oriented sexual encounter as opposed to anonymous sex.

Consider Wendy, a thirty-six-year-old teacher and wife of a university professor. She reports spending about fifteen hours per week for the past two years in Internet chat rooms. This time was previously spent on her work, husband, and three children. Her pattern has been to meet men online and then arrange for an offline encounter with them at hotels or other locations, for the express purpose of having sex. She describes her addiction cycle as follows:

> First I would make up an excuse to leave the house. Then I'd start down my list of potential partners till I found a local guy who was available at the same time I was. I would lie to my spouse and family and go out to meet him. I'd have sex with him and sometimes talk for a few minutes. After the sex, I'd return home as if nothing had happened.

Nonetheless, her own words reveal that what she really wants is to be loved by an exciting man:

> I start to get attached emotionally and it scares the men off; they just want free sex. I can't seem to have a meaningful relationship. . . . Usually we just have sex. A few have been actual relationships, but they never lasted more than a month. . . . I have shut down all my normal emotions and just deal with things unrealistically, such as imagining that one day one of these men will really love me. I shut out the hurt I feel each time a relationship doesn't work out. I repeatedly ignore my family when they need me, in order to talk online.

Wendy's husband, Ted, found out about her sexual acting out eight months earlier when she forgot to turn off her computer after planning online to meet another man. When Ted came home shortly after her departure, he read her e-mail correspondence and figured out what was up. In Ted's confrontation of Wendy when she returned, she confessed not only to that meeting, but also to having had sex with several other men. Wendy cried and said she knew she had a serious problem, but that the person she really loved was Ted. She promised to get help, and Ted believed her. Since then, she has been more careful to cover her tracks.

Ted, a quiet, introverted man ten years older than Wendy, couldn't believe his good luck twelve years earlier when she agreed to marry him. At his university, Ted is a caring professor who spends long hours at his office doing research and helping students with their advanced math problems. Although he feels uncomfortable expressing his emotions, he cannot imagine life without Wendy, on whom he is very dependent. Ted has chosen to stay with his wife, but in the past eight months he has been so depressed that his doctor has put him on Prozac. This medication has improved Ted's mood and has allowed him to continue functioning well at work, but it has also decreased his sex drive, a common side effect.

Wendy describes Ted as a caring person who is trying his best to help her. When asked what is missing in their marriage and what she is looking for online, Wendy replied:

> I love my husband very much and want to stay with him. He loves me to the best of his ability, but for some reason it never seems to be what I need physically, emotionally, or spiritually. . . . I want to be accepted and loved by someone who will be my hero. I know that is not really going to happen, but I keep looking anyway. I haven't bottomed out yet. Why don't I make some real changes? Maybe because I am afraid of being alone, without someone to play with. I love the

attention, the men's letters and phone calls, etc. I also crave the sex. I seem to be unable to say no. I place myself in situations that just have a direct path to sex.

Wendy, like many sex addicts, experienced abuse and emotional abandonment in childhood. Often, survivors of childhood abuses (physical, emotional, and/or sexual) confuse sex with love and caring and tend to use sexualized ways of relating to others to affirm their own true value and worth as people. In childhood, these abuse victims were powerless over what they did or did not get. Many survivors of childhood abuse and abandonment later come to believe that sex, flirtation, and seduction can give them power and enable them to get the love and attention they did not receive as children, without making themselves vulnerable to rejection or loss. As adult survivors and sex addicts themselves, they attempt to use sex to acquire power and a sense of being desired. These dysfunctional attempts to meet deeper emotional needs are now frequently activated through the Internet.

The availability and convenience of the Internet provides a nearly instantaneous means of accomplishing these goals, but at a very high cost. Internet romance keeps addicts searching for love and validation, but often finding only more pain and sometimes danger.

Although women usually favor relational activities over straight porn, some women cybersex users do get hooked on visual images. Yvonne is single and twenty-nine years old and spends several hours a week online viewing hard-core pornographic photos including those showing sadomasochistic (S&M) activities. Yvonne says:

The material that is written for women is usually in the "love addiction" realm and not straight sex addiction. There are women out there like myself who are aroused visually like men and have some characteristics that more closely follow typical male sex addiction. I don't have sex to appease the man in my life or get his love; I have sex for the rush of orgasm, for the medication.

Compared with men, women cybersex and romance addicts face additional challenges when they seek help:

- increased shame about the activities
- less societal acceptance of women's sexual (and cyber-sexual) behaviors
- fewer support group meetings where women feel comfortable
- lack of knowledge by therapists about cybersex in general and about women's activities in particular

The remaining chapters focus on how both men and women can get help and how they can facilitate their recovery from cybersex addiction.

FIVE

The Cybersex Widow(er)

▣ ▣ ▣

When does cybersex and cyber-romance cross the line and violate the integrity of a committed relationship? How is cybersex really cheating? After all, many people wonder, what's the fuss? It's not really an affair and you can't catch a sexually transmitted disease. So, what's the big deal? When someone in a committed relationship becomes more involved in computer sex, flirtation, and romantic intrigues than in making love with his or her live partner, there are significant consequences for their relationship. We asked women and men who felt they had lost their partners (emotionally, intellectually, physically, and spiritually) to cybersex to tell us in their own words how this affected them. One hundred people—ninety-seven women and three men—responded to an online survey and wrote us about their reactions.[1] This chapter explores their responses and what they taught us about living with a cybersex addict.

SEX AND THE PRIMARY RELATIONSHIP

Consider Elena, thirty-eight, who is in the process of divorcing her husband after a fifteen-year marriage:

> I knew my husband was masturbating all the time, but I
> thought it was my fault, that I just wasn't attractive enough for

him. When I found pornography files on his computer going back five years, everything made sense. I had been in denial about how much I knew and how much my life was out of control. I feel very used and violated because of this behavior, and I have lost my trust.

My husband would blame me when I would catch him masturbating at the computer. He would not do any chores when I was out; when I returned, he would clear the computer screen and turn off the light really fast. He would keep looking at his pants to see if I could tell he had an erection. He would run out of the bedroom like he was just changing. At other times, he would call me and say he was coming right home at four o'clock, and not show up until three hours later, or he would say he was working really hard and not to give him a hard time.

I knew he would masturbate if I left the house. I never said no to sex unless I was not feeling well or I was working. I believed that if I had sex more often, or if I were better at sex, he would not masturbate as much. I surveyed my friends to see if they'd caught their husbands masturbating, to see how often they thought it was normal to masturbate, to see what kind of sex they had with their husbands and how often.

I thought I was not good enough because I did not look like the girls in the computer pictures. I thought if I dressed and looked better, it would keep him interested. Eventually, I gave up competing with his masturbating and chose not to have sex with him. I would not walk into the room at night because I did not want to walk in on him.

If the kids and I were coming home and his car was in the driveway, I would run into the house first and be loud so the kids would not walk in on him masturbating. I found semen on my office chair and lubricant next to the keyboard. I stopped making dinner because I would not know when he'd be coming home. I would have to mentally prepare myself for sex because it got so I didn't want it. At times, I would get dressed fast so he wouldn't see my body and want to have sex with me. I tried to talk with him many times about masturbation and how often he expected to have sex with me. I was in denial about how unhappy I was.

My husband believes he does not have a problem. He feels it's no big deal since he claims he is being faithful to me. He thinks all he needs is a more accepting wife.

Without fully understanding the intensity of the cybersex experience, it would be easy to assume that people are attracted to Internet pornography because they are not getting enough "good sex" at home. Some partners of cybersex addicts also make the same erroneous assumption. When in fact they do have an exciting sexual relationship with the cybersex user, they are confused. For example, Alexis, thirty-one, who has been married only a year, wrote:

When I know that my husband has masturbated to cyberporn, I don't want him to touch me. I feel like leftovers, not first-run as I should be. My self-esteem is damaged beyond belief. To be honest, our sex life has always been pretty incredible—we are not prudes by any means. I just don't understand. How can it be *soooo* good for both of us but still not enough for him?

IS IT REALLY CHEATING?

With the advent of digital video-streaming, images can be captured and sent, and responses returned, all in real time. As the technology of the Internet has advanced, the experience of cybersex and cyber-romance has gone beyond still photos and words into live-action images and on-demand responses. The partner's pain and confusion is multiplied if the cybersex addict engages in real-time online sex with another person. One distraught woman wrote the following:

> My husband is using sexual energy that should be used with me. The person on the other end of that computer is live and is participating in a sexual activity with him. They are doing it together and responding to each other. It is one thing to masturbate to a two-dimensional screen image. But to engage in an interactive sexual encounter means that you are being sexual with another person, and that is cheating.

Extensive cybersex involvement by one partner can harm the entire family. The resulting problems come to affect the partner's feelings, the couple's sexual relationship, and other family members.

Effects on the Partner's Emotional State

Most partners described some combination of devastation, hurt, betrayal, loss of self-esteem, abandonment, mistrust, suspicion, fear, and a lack of intimacy in their relationship. Two partners reported actually having become physically abusive to their husbands, hitting them and throwing objects at them. Other reactions include feeling sexually inadequate, unattractive, and even ugly; doubting one's judgment or sanity; or experiencing severe depression. Two women in the survey reported that they were hospitalized for suicide attempts.

The lies associated with cybersex activities were a major cause of distress for the partners. One woman wrote, "The lies he told me concerning his whereabouts, while looking me straight in the eye, have hurt worse than his out-of-control sexual behavior." Despite the cybersex user's repeated promises to stop, the behavior would continue, often with increased lying and secrecy. With each discovery, trust was further eroded. The partners' self-esteem plummeted, and they felt betrayed and rejected. Some partners described a predominant fear that the Internet activities would resume; others primarily experienced feelings of anger.

A thirty-six-year-old woman, married five years, reported:

> I blamed myself for his problem and felt inadequate—not attractive enough, not adventurous enough, etc.—confused about whether this was something I was imagining, or did I have hang-ups about sex? How could I trust or believe him when he would continually lie to me even in the face of reality when I caught him in the act? He would try to make me feel guilty and often succeeded.

A fifty-five-year-old woman, married thirty-six years, described her range of feelings:

> His behavior has left me feeling alone, isolated, rejected, and less than a desired woman. Masturbation hangs a sign on the door that says, "You are not needed. I can take care of myself, thank you very much." I have threatened, manipulated, tried to control, cried, gave him the cold shoulder, yelled, tried to be understanding, and even tried to ignore it.

The cybersex user's perspective was described by a twenty-nine-year-old man, with no history of compulsive sexual behaviors, who in the year following the purchase of a computer became caught up in a rapidly progressive addiction:

> Emotionally I was in a daze for that whole year of being online. I was occasionally there to support my wife, but I seemed always to be thinking about the next time I could get online and when my next day off from work would be. Sometimes my wife would ask me to pick her up for lunch and I'd get angry, lying about errands I had to do, so I could stay home

and surf the Net. Our relationship became significantly strained. We'd go months without having sex. My wife said she felt extremely alone during that period.

Is Virtual or Real Sex Better?

Knowing that the cybersex addict's head is full of sexual images and fantasy, many partners can't help comparing themselves with the online fantasy person in terms of appearance, desirability, and repertoire of sexual behaviors. Both cybersex addicts and partners make such comparisons. Partners feel that they are competing with the computer images and people. ("If only I was perfect like his porn women, then he would want the real thing and love me." "How can I compete with hundreds of anonymous men who are now in our bed?") The result is often confusion: on the one hand, a desire to emulate and be as desirable as the cyber-image, and on the other hand, revulsion at the lack of intimacy and mechanical nature of the sex. Survey respondents reported vacillating between these two polarities.

A thirty-eight-year-old woman, divorcing after a fifteen-year marriage, confided:

> I thought I was not good enough because I did not look like the girls in the pictures. I thought that if I dressed and looked good, it would keep him interested. Then I'd give up on competing with his masturbating and not want to have sex with him at all.

Indeed, many cyberporn addicts do come to prefer virtual sex with fantasy women or men rather than real-life sex with their partners, so the partners' fears and concerns are often justified. A fifty-eight-year-old man wrote, "My sex life with my wife became totally unfulfilling and I no longer felt closeness or intimacy with her." According to a forty-five-year-old man, "I was so into meeting new fit, good-looking women online that I spent less sexual time with my wife and wasn't as turned on by her."

THE EFFECT ON THE
SEXUAL RELATIONSHIP

Two-thirds of the survey respondents described sexual problems in the couple relationship resulting from the cybersex involvement. In some cases the sexual problems resulted in decreased interest by the cybersex user in couple sex. In others, it was the partner who lost interest, and in some cases both partners were less interested in sex with each other. Overall, in only 30 percent of the relationships were both partners still interested in sex with each other. Partners of the cybersex users felt objectified, compared themselves unfavorably with the cybersex partners, initially attempted to increase the quantity or variety of sexual activities, and subsequently experienced a decreased frequency of sexual relations with the cybersex addict. In 20 percent of the cases, both partners lost interest in couple sex. Among these couples, the cybersex addict was more interested in sex with the computer than with the spouse. In turn, the spouse felt angry, rejected, and unable to compete.

Three of the ninety-seven female survey respondents reported having their own extramarital affairs or encounters, either to shore up their self-esteem or to get revenge on their spouses. One of them, a thirty-five-year-old nurse who'd been married eleven years, wrote:

We had almost no sex life at all. I was tired of carrying the entire burden of trying to make our relationship work. It got so bad at one point that I began to believe my marriage was over. I started looking around for someone to talk to online. One day in the hospital I ran into a man I'd had a crush on many years before, when I was a nursing student. He had recently moved back to our community after getting a divorce. We went to the cafeteria for coffee and had several other meetings, and eventually I had a one-night stand with him. My husband was so wrapped up in his addiction that he suspected nothing.

A thirty-four-year-old woman who had learned of her husband's intense cybersex involvement only weeks earlier, described the effects on the couple's sexual relationship:

I realize now that many of the things he most liked and requested when we made love were re-creations of downloaded images. He is no longer able to be intimate. He objectifies me, other women, and girls on the streets. When we're together in bed, he fantasizes about the women he's seen online and imagines that he's having sex with one of them. I feel humiliated, used, betrayed, lied to, and misled. It's almost impossible to let him touch me without feeling really yucky. I tried to continue being sexual with him initially. In fact, I tried being "more" sexual, to compete better with the porn girls, but I couldn't do it. Now we just stopped having sex altogether.

When the Cybersex User Loses Interest in Sex with the Real-Life Partner

In one-third of the survey cases the cybersex user was no longer interested in sex. The willing partner reported that the addict made excuses like not being in the mood, being too tired, working too hard, that the children might hear, that his or her back hurts too much, or that he or she would have already climaxed and not want sex. In these cases, during couple sex, some of these addicts appeared distant, emotionally detached, and interested only in their own pleasure. The partner ended up doing most or all of the initiating, either to get her or his own needs met, or in an attempt to get the addict to decrease the online activities. The addict often blamed the partner for the couple's sexual problems. In some cases the partner was asked to participate in sexual activities that she or he found objectionable. A thirty-three-year-old gay man in a committed relationship with a cybersex addict reported:

> Currently my partner and I have sex once every three months, usually only after I get mad, and I suppose he ends up feeling obligated. Although I know that I am bright and attractive, emotionally I feel ugly, worthless, and unwanted by him or anybody else. For me the issue has not been the difference between him having computer sex or actual physical contact. It is that someone else is receiving his attention and I am not. I do many mental gymnastics in order to cope with this. To prevent becoming irritated with my partner because he rejects my sexual advances, I masturbate daily with the hope that it will prevent me from becoming "horny." Sometimes it works. I would not care at all if he masturbated online with a host of others, as long as I remained an active part of his love life.

A forty-five-year-old man, who spent much time masturbating to online pictures of nude women, explained:

> My sexual energy was "saved" for the Internet. I lost interest in sex with my wife because I knew there were an unlimited number of photos on the Net that could "get me off" any time I preferred.

When the Partner Alone Loses Interest in Couple Sex

Some partners in the survey felt so repelled and disgusted by the cybersex addict's online or real sexual activities that they no longer wanted to have sex. Others could no longer tolerate the addict's detachment and lack of emotional connection during sex. Some spouses lost sexual interest because they were too angry about the addict's denial that there was a problem. Other partners felt angry, repelled, used, objectified, or "like a prostitute" because of the cybersex addict's pressure or requests for them to dress in certain ways or perform new sexual acts. In 40 percent of the one hundred relationships described in the survey, the partners were aware that the cybersex addict had also had offline sexual affairs. Some of the significant others subsequently avoided sex with the addict out of fear of catching a disease, or because the addicted partner had already caught a disease.

A forty-four-year-old accountant, married twenty-six years to a female sex addict who was his childhood sweetheart, is still in the relationship. He is aware that his wife is still involved in cybersex activities. He has had some therapy but is still working through his anger and depression. He wrote:

> At first we had sex more than ever, as I desperately tried to prove myself; then sex with her made me sick. I get strong pictures of what she did and lusted after, and then I get repelled and feel bad. I used to see sex as a very intimate, loving thing. We always had a lot of sex, and I felt we were intimate. Since I found out my wife was not on the same page, I can't be intimate or vulnerable—sex is now more recreational or just out of need.

A forty-nine-year-old woman, who has been married for nine years to her second husband, describes how initially they had a frequent and enjoyable sexual relationship, but for the past three years sex has been infrequent and perfunctory. She described her dissatisfaction:

> Sometimes I would "take sex" from him because I felt he owed me that much. But basically any sex that occurred was unsatisfying and left me feeling angry, unwanted, unattractive, and used. Now I don't feel anything when we are sexual. I can no longer reach an orgasm with him. I'm always afraid that any sexual attention he gives me is because he's been viewing cyberporn or talking sexual with someone online. It makes it hard to just enjoy the here and now with him.

Some women became frustrated when their male partners considered their cybersex involvement to be typical of any "normal, healthy male" and were unwilling to acknowledge that their sexual behavior was harming the relationship. The frustration often turned to anger, and the anger led to a loss of interest in the couple's sexual relationship.

Will More Real-Life Sex Help?

It is still a common notion that a person who fears his or her spouse's roving eye while he or she is out of town should provide a night of lovemaking before departure. The mistaken belief is that good sex at home will prevent straying while away. In reality, the allure of illicit sex with an unfamiliar partner can survive even abundant sex at home with a willing but familiar mate. This same false logic is applied by many partners who are aware of the cybersex addict's involvement with Internet sex. Some partners either increase the frequency of sexual activities with the cybersex user, or else agree to participate in sexual activities with which they may be uncomfortable or that they find offensive.

A thirty-nine-year-old woman, married eight years but now divorced, wrote the following:

> I tried to initiate a variety of things I saw in *Penthouse*. I feel ashamed about the activities I've suggested, which I thought would change his behavior. I have to remind myself every day that that wasn't my normal behavior. I am trying to forgive myself. It's extremely difficult.

Some partners reluctantly decide to join the addict in cybersex activities. Like the following thirty-four-year-old woman, who'd been married for fourteen years, they usually learn that their involvement in these activities does not prevent the cybersex addict from continuing to engage in cybersex with others:

> My husband is a minister who was stationed overseas for a year. We chatted daily, but never sexually. One day he admitted to me that he'd been involved in cybersex activities with other women online. He said it had nothing to do with us and that it didn't affect his feelings for me. I felt cheated. Why wouldn't he ask *me* to have cybersex? I guessed it was because he thought I was too old-fashioned, so I told him I was willing to try it with him. I wasn't comfortable with this, but I thought I could "rescue" him. We began a cybersex relationship. But much to my horror, he never quit with all the anonymous partners. Instead he lumped me together with all the online whores. When he returned, he continued his cybersex even though we were reunited. We're still together, but his online activities have really come between us.

Attempts to solve the cybersex problem by providing more real-life sex are usually ineffective and are mostly short-lived. It's common for partners who participated in activities with which they were uncomfortable to later feel shame and anger.

Trying to control the cybersex addict's behavior and get his or her attention is usually unsuccessful.

WHAT'S THE BIG DEAL ABOUT ONLINE SEX?

Some Internet pornography addicts never leave the solitude of their fantasy computer world; others use the Internet as a gateway to real sexual encounters with other people. To help readers understand why marriages and long-term relationships break up even though cybersex doesn't involve skin-to-skin contact, people who experienced this situation were asked to present their viewpoint in the survey. Here were the most common reasons for such breakups:

- a concern about escalation of the behaviors
- the belief that a cybersex affair is still cheating
- the effect on the partner's self-esteem
- the effect on the marriage and children

Each of these reasons will be examined in more detail in the pages that follow.

Concern about Escalation

One of the common features of all addictions is increasing tolerance to the substance or behavior being used. In other words, the addict has to do more and more over time to get the same level of excitement. Online viewing, which begins as harmless recreation, can become an all-consuming activity, taking the user away from family and work. It can also lead to offline sexual encounters with those met online or even a need for real-life sexual activities that aren't computer related.

According to the survey respondents, 40 percent of the cyber-sex addicts had also engaged in offline sexual activities. This surely is an underestimate, since it is likely that not all partners were aware of such behaviors.

Some cybersex users describe a progression of their addiction. A thirty-two-year-old man with a prior history of compulsive sexual behaviors wrote:

> Cybersex really accelerated my addiction. It went from just pornographic magazines and movies, to spending hours on end on the computer looking at images, and finally to many hours chatting with anyone who would engage in sexual "talk" with me. It took only three months to go from simple e-mail correspondence to all this. Had my wife not found a porn disk in my disk drive, it would have only been a matter of time before I started to meet women in person. Considering my shyness and preference of fantasy over being with real women, meeting a live woman would have been a big step!

Describing the activities of her husband, whose business often took him away from home, a forty-one-year-old divorced woman related her story:

> My husband's compulsive sexual activities quickly progressed. He first got into print pornography, then real-time cybersex that led to phone sex. Next he answered personals and placed his own ads when out of town. This evolved into his placing an ad in porno sites for group sex and discreet affairs. He's had multiple partners. He deceives women by telling them that he's single and lives in the town he's due to work in.

In other cases, no live sexual encounters occurred with people the addict met online, but the computer sexual activity did trigger other offline addictive behaviors. One gay man wrote that since being online, his partner had begun to go out and have anonymous sex. Women wrote that their partners had begun new activities, such as visiting a sexual massage parlor, hiring prostitutes, having the first offline affair, or having additional affairs.

On the Internet it is possible to find groups of people who are interested in all kinds of unusual or even deviant sexual practices. Interacting with these people helps to desensitize the user and "normalizes" these activities. Some cybersex users eventually blame their partners for their relationship problems, citing their unwillingness to engage in these behaviors. Even if the viewers' activity never goes beyond traditional pornography, prolonged cybersex activities can negatively affect the viewer, as this thirty-year-old unmarried man discovered about himself:

> Throughout the last couple of years, the more porn I've viewed, the less sensitive I am to porn that I used to find offensive. Now I get turned on by some of it (anal sex, women peeing, etc.). The sheer quantity of porn on the Net has done this. It's so easy to click on these things out of curiosity in the privacy of your own home. The more you view, the less sensitized you become. I used to be only into soft-core porn showing the beauty of the female form. Now I'm into explicit hard-core.

Cybersex Is Still Cheating

To the 30 percent of the survey respondents who considered online sexual activities the same as adultery, the lying and emotional unavailability of their partner felt the same as a real affair would. Many partners felt that the lies, which are often the most painful part of a real-life affair, were just as excruciating for partners involved in cybersex. They felt betrayed, devalued, deceived, "less than," and abandoned—the same as with a real affair. They mourned the loss of the sexual intimacy they previously had with their spouse. One woman wrote, "I may not be getting a disease from him, but I'm not getting anything else either!" In real-life affairs, it is hard for the spouse to compete with the excitement of the affair partner. Similarly, with cybersex, the spouse is competing with idealized fantasy partners who are always available, make no demands, and are willing to do whatever the cybersex addict wants. The pain is increased when the addict has real-time online sex with another person. Most partners agreed that, except for the absent risk of sexually transmitted diseases, real-time online sex is definitely the same as being unfaithful.

Finally, many survey respondents complained that cybersex took their partner away from the relationship itself. The resulting emotional detachment was viewed as a real loss by the partner. A thirty-nine-year-old woman, married fourteen years, explained:

> He did have affairs, although not physically. He had affairs of the mind, and that to me is as much a violation as if he actually had a physical affair with someone. According to my religious beliefs, he committed adultery just the same as if he had another real partner. Moreover, in one sense I feel that having an affair of the mind is worse than having an actual partner. My husband can, at any time, have an "affair" without leaving the house or seeing another human being.

The 40 percent of the spouses who knew about their partner's real-life extramarital sexual encounters were able to compare how they felt about their partner's cybersex activities against how they felt about their live affairs. Several experienced the same hurt. A thirty-eight-year-old woman, married eighteen years, anguished:

They should try it for themselves one time, and see how it feels to be less important to their partner than a picture on a computer screen! They should see what it feels like to lie in bed and know their partner is on the computer and what he is doing with it. It's not going to do much for their self-esteem. My husband has actually cheated on me with a real partner, and it *feels no different!* The online "safe" cheating feels to me just as dirty and filthy as does the "real-life" cheating.

Cybersex Destroys the Partner's Self-Esteem

Compulsive cybersex can tap into a partner's deepest insecurities about his or her ability to measure up. The need to compete with interactive online sex pressures the partner into unwanted sexual activities. "Fantasy sex leaves practically nothing to be desired when compared with the all-too-human and flawed spouse," explained one woman. Another woman wondered: "When he closes his eyes when we are together, what is he thinking of? The babe on the screen? Is he happy with my body? Is he grossed out?"

Even the best-adjusted person is likely to feel bad when repeatedly seeing his or her spouse preferring solitary sex with a computer screen to flesh-and-blood lovemaking. A thirty-seven-year-old woman, married ten years, explained:

True, you don't have the risk of the diseases, but it is still an emotional thing. It's hard to think that sex addicts want to do it without the actual human touch of another—how can it be better for them? Especially since they have to do all the work themselves! Plus, when the sex addict is having couple sex with you, they are not really there emotionally. They are thinking about and picturing the "others" that they were with, what they were saying to them, etc. In reality, the sex addict is getting off on something that has nothing to do with you. It really hurts your self-esteem, and most of us don't have a very good self-esteem to begin with.

Harm to Primary Relationship and to Children

Even when partners did not view the cybersex activities as an affair, the addict's Internet use was considered a major contributor to discord in the relationship. The time involvement, the emotional distancing, the deception, and the arguments begun by addicts to justify time away from the family all negatively impacted marriages.

For a person in a committed relationship, cybersex activities can escalate relationship conflict. A parent's cybersex involvement can also negatively impact the children. Most commonly, this is because the cybersex addict's activities take time away from being a parent. Addicts often go through the motions of parenting without the emotional interactions needed to help children feel bonded and attached. Spouses may also be unavailable for parenting because of their preoccupation with the addict's sexual activities. In cases where parents divorce, the children lose the presence of a parent in the home. Even in marriages that remain intact, the children often witness arguments, conflict, and stress in the home. In some cases, the children actually come upon and view the pornography or witness a parent masturbating at the computer. Some children found pornography that had been left on the computer, had walked in when the cybersex addict was chatting in a chat room, had overheard the addict having phone sex, or had observed the addict having interactive sex online. Several mothers were worried because their husbands surfed the Net while supposedly baby-sitting young children. Sometimes these children were exposed to the pornography and masturbation. In some families, teenage children began viewing online pornography themselves.

Testimonials from spouses and partners, such as those presented in this chapter, can help the reader more fully understand the effects of Internet sex addiction on the family, even when real-life affairs are not present.

SIX

Doing the Work: Making a Plan for Cybersex Recovery

■   ■   ■

Recovery from any addiction is a simple process to define, but not always easy to carry out. The simple part of the process lies in outlining and organizing the steps toward stopping the problem behavior. Addicts are given instructions about what to do and what not to do and are told that if they follow these steps, things will get better. Developing a commitment to following that plan of action *no matter what* is the more difficult aspect of creating change. It is not difficult to find the process that promotes healing; the hard part is getting addicted people to become willing to follow through consistently. Cybersex addicts can clearly learn that certain Internet activities are simply off-limits. However, understanding the issues can mean little when they are alone one afternoon and are faced with porn-related e-mail. It takes discipline and practice to continue to avoid these situations on a regular basis.

The real problem lies in the mind of the addicted person who, like anyone else, wants to rely on his or her own judgment in making decisions. Unfortunately, people who are addicted to substances or behaviors suffer from faulty and distorted thinking, particularly in the area of their addictive behavior patterns. When confronted with what would seem to someone else to be a simple choice regarding problem behavior, an addict's common sense often goes out the window, quickly replaced by an incorrect but more exciting decision. In the words of one cybersex addict:

> I made so many promises to myself to stop looking at sex online. Promises to myself, promises to my lover. Some of the time it seemed really easy, and I felt good about my ability to stay away from it. Other days, when I was feeling stressed or distracted, it seems like no matter what I did, I would end up right back in those chat rooms.

Seeing a counselor familiar with addiction and attending self-help meetings can help motivate cybersex addicts to create and follow a recovery plan that makes them accountable for their ongoing recovery. The following section describes some elements of a personal program of change and recovery for the cybersex addict. Some people may need additional elements. These are best developed with the assistance of a knowledgeable counselor, therapist, or another person who has successfully worked on these issues.

People truly addicted to computer sex, whether online or off-, have to determine when, how, and under what circumstances they will again be able to use the computer for non-sexual purposes. Making declarations such as "I will never go to X-rated sites again!" or "I will never get involved in another chat line" are not generally strong enough statements for addicts to hold onto when in a challenging moment. Some cybersex addicts will simply not be able to go online again at all, or at least for a specific period of time. For example, those in relationships may find that it is too painful for the spouse or partner to see them once again online at the computer. For others, any online use may inevitably lead to sexual acting out, and they must remain offline indefinitely.

Whatever the eventual outcome, it is a good idea in the first few weeks of recovery to entirely avoid online use. A gradual return to online use may be acceptable once certain ground rules are established and support is in place. Initially, the best way to stay offline is simply to disconnect the modem or direct service line. It may be necessary to put the computer in another location or give it to a friend for safekeeping. Often, simply stating, "Now I am going to stay offline" isn't enough, particularly for those who are so strongly tempted to "just take a quick look at that Web site that used to be so hot." Some period of complete disconnection may be essential in early recovery. This was the solution for the man who wrote:

> Although I really did feel committed to staying out of my sexual problem areas, it was so easy to just pop into a chat room to see who was there. I seemed to have endless reasons to have to be online, and once there, the porn sites were just a single link away. I couldn't seem to stay out of it. Sometimes I would think everything was fine, only to find myself opening unsolicited sexual e-mails and clicking my way right back to where I started.

First and foremost, cybersex addicts cannot truly change their behavior by themselves. The very nature of addiction implies that addicts suffer from a kind of distorted thinking; therefore, recovery often requires both the insight and accountability that others can provide. Unfortunately, spouses and partners are usually not the best people to turn to as primary resources for the recovery process. No matter how well intentioned they may be, the issues are too painful and close to home for most addict's partners to be objective. The best people to provide support and guidance are those with similar problems who are in the process of getting better. These people can most readily be found in Twelve Step sexual recovery programs (see appendix 1) and through therapists and professionals who specialize in sexual addiction. Having a prepared list of such outsiders often proves critical when the recovering addict is close to relapse and needs to call or otherwise reach out to someone for support, as the following story illustrates:

> It felt too shameful to turn to my lover for support when I wanted to go online. I just knew that he would end up blaming himself or feeling inadequate no matter how much he wanted to help. It only really got better when I found people who weren't so directly affected by my problem. They were able to be my reality check when I needed someone who could understand.

Second, to create change, the addict must honestly acknowledge that a real problem exists. That problem might be defined as the effect that the cybersex behavior has had on others. When the addict accepts that he or she has a behavior problem, the natural resistance to following the steps to recovery begins to break down. Even a grudging willingness and superficial understanding of the addiction is a start.

A WORD ON SEX ADDICTION

Some cybersex addicts find themselves addicted purely to the intensity and arousal provided through computer sex. Others may discover, while exploring these issues, that they have a propensity for addictive sexual behaviors in general. In addition to the problems generated by online sexual use, longer-term problems with addictive sexual behaviors may be identified. Many discover through writing and self-examination that they were involved in phone sex before or they became "hooked" on cybersex activities. A previous history of addictive use of masturbation to porn videos and magazines often accompanies cybersex addiction. Some people acted out sexually with anonymous partners, with prostitutes, and by obtaining "sensual" massages. Still others constantly find themselves objectifying and sexualizing everyone they see. In the early stages of change, it is not unusual for a cybersex addict to recognize and own up to long histories of hidden and secretive sexual lives extending far beyond the computer. As addicts progress in their recovery, avoiding these compulsive sexual behaviors will need to be incorporated into an overall plan to address sexual recovery. For more help, see G-SAST (the Male Sexual Addiction Screening Test) and the list of Twelve Step recovery programs in appendix 1.

FIRST STEPS FOR THE CYBERSEX ADDICT

The following are specific steps that can lead addicts away from the immediate temptations and distractions of their online behavior:

1. Start by going through your computer files and computer history while being monitored by a safe someone else *in the room*. Look through all "downloaded" files and old mail for pictures or attachments, often found as GIF or JPEG files. Use the computer's "find files" search ability to look for items with the words *sex, porn, photo*, and so on. Delete *all* files with sexual or romantic content—letters, photos, e-mail, sexual jokes, and pornography. The other person is nearby as a support. That person will ensure that mail is not longingly reread, old photos glanced at, or online relationships re-engaged. There is no need to review this stuff; just

get rid of it! It is important to remember to delete all online mail saved in the "personal filing cabinet," files which are automatically saved for you by the various Internet service providers (ISPs) such as America Online (AOL), CompuServe, and Earthlink. If you have trouble finding this online history, contact your ISP and ask them how it can be obtained. Remove any history of past contacts and favorite Web sites and newsgroups. Don't forget the e-mail address book! This process should be followed on both personal and work computers.

Although it is not generally recommended that the addict's spouse or partner be the person to monitor the addict's computer cleanup or ongoing use, in early recovery this may be the most convenient person for the task.

2. Write or phone any membership porn companies and ask to have your membership canceled and for charges on your credit card to discontinue. If necessary, ask your credit card company to cancel that particular card and issue you a new number.

3. Delete any screen name used online for sexual or romantic contact. Screen names can be changed or deleted through the various online service companies. Most offer instructions on how to accomplish this through their online "help" or member support areas.

4. Delete any saved files that could be used toward sexual acting out. These could include written self-descriptions or self-photos that may have evaded deletion while doing step one.

5. Remove any live video equipment from the computer (at least for a period of time). This will be helpful in avoiding easy access to this type of interactive activity.

6. Utilize any blocking services offered by your Internet provider. Earthlink, AOL, and other ISPs have blocking services or parental controls that can help eliminate sexually oriented material or whole subject areas from being received along with unsolicited mail from former online sexual or romantic partners. Specific e-mail addresses and Web sites can be blocked from communication. These blocking services can be accessed through Keyword: Parental Control or by accessing "Help" through the ISP.

7. Get rid of any pornography or sexually interactive stories purchased on compact disc or stored previously on a floppy disk.

At Home

In some homes, maintaining online use of the computer is necessary for various reasons. Some examples are maintaining a home office or using the Internet to book plane tickets, do research, or for children to work online for school. If you or a family member needs to continue using the computer online, here are some simple, helpful guidelines:

1. *Purchase blocking software.* Blocking software designed to eliminate access to sexual content and other specific types of sites can be purchased and downloaded over the Internet or in computer stores. This software, which will provide a screen for 90 percent of the problem sites, is a *must-have* for cybersex addicts who intend to use the Internet again. Although with enough effort, the software can be defeated, it provides the cybersex addict with time to reflect before logging on to an inappropriate site. It is essential when loading this software to *give the access code to someone else* (preferably someone

else in cybersex recovery—not a spouse or partner). Without the access code, it's impossible to remove the blocking software. Specific examples of blocking programs are SurfWatch, Net Nanny, and Cyber Patrol.

2. *Move the computer.* Isolation and the potential for getting away with illicit actions feed the addiction. Cybersex addicts who live with others should not keep their home computer in an isolated location. Moving it to a family room or other public area can help partners feel less suspicious and uncomfortable, and it keeps temptations away.

3. *Go online only when someone else is home.* Accountability is established by having others around.

4. *Change online providers.* Several online Internet service providers (ISPs) offer access only to sites that their evaluation team has deemed appropriate for children and families. Such providers exclude sexual-content sites.

5. *Go online for e-mail only.* If there is no reason to be searching online, don't. Make a written and verbal commitment to avoid any online searching or activity. Let others gather information or data if that becomes necessary.

6. *Create online accountability.* One of the keys to any successful recovery program is to use others for support. Make it a habit when going online to call a friend first, or better yet, someone from a support group—this is called bookending. By making a commitment to another person to stay out of problem online sites and calling that person back when offline, accountability is created.

7. *Write a commitment for change.* Many people attempting change will make verbal commitments to themselves or others outlining what they will no longer do. It is better

to document the commitment in the form of a signed and witnessed contract. Making an agreement in writing and having it signed and witnessed by a spouse, therapist, or Twelve Step support person goes a long way toward ensuring implementation of a solid commitment (see "Creating a Sexual Recovery Plan" later in the chapter, on page 120).

8. *Make a commitment to honesty.* Ending the lying to self and others is the most profound part of the recovery process. Addicts truly take their most important recovery step by making a decision to end deceit, dishonesty, and a double life.

In the Workplace

When addicts act out by going to sexual-content or relationship sites while at work, they are likely to be embarrassed, be written up, or lose a valued job. Most companies have now adopted a zero-tolerance policy for such behavior in the workplace. When the latest e-mail joke or an employee's baby picture is being "passed" around the office, company policies are often easily forgotten or minimized. The cybersex addict may think, Everyone is looking at something personal on their computer, what's the big deal? But sexual activity in the workplace *is* a big deal. Many cybersex addicts try to avoid being observed by staying late to access sexual content, unaware that in the workplace they are often continuously monitored when online. Every site and piece of mail accessed from an individual workstation has the potential to be detected by management through networked systems and programs that follow a user's path as he or she traverses the Internet.

By the time they formulate a recovery plan, some cybersex addicts have already used the office computer to access online sexual material. Even if the addict has used only the home computer for cybersex purposes, the office computer constitutes a significant risk for recovering cybersex addicts. If online work in the office is a necessity, the following steps may be helpful:

1. *Remove any files* or history of past sexual activity from the computer. (See step one on pages 113–114 of this chapter.) Ask another knowledgeable recovering person for help in removing information from the hard drive.
2. *Move the position of the computer screen.* If your office computer screen faces away from people walking by or entering your workstation, move the screen so that others can view what is being accessed or worked on.
3. *If possible, install blocking software* on a work PC. In a non-networked system this should be a fairly simple task. (See item one, pages 115–116).
4. *Go online only during work hours.* Don't stay late to work on projects and take on assignments involving Internet use. Avoid being alone in the office.
5. *If possible, find a safe person in the workplace to turn to for help when needed.* Obviously, it may not be wise to reveal to your boss a history of sexually acting out at work, unless you've been caught. You can recruit others for support and help, however. Ask co-workers whom you trust to go out for coffee breaks, walks, and to just sit and talk. It may be appropriate to at least disclose that valuable work time is being taken up by being "obsessive" on the Internet and that you need some support.
6. *Take breaks when feeling tempted.* Go for therapeutic walks. Get out of your workstation. Find a quiet place to do some meditating or some breathing exercises. A little time and distance goes a long way toward avoiding old behavior.

7. *Use the telephone.* Call other people to check in for support during the workday.
8. *Display inspirational photos* around the computer screen. Family photos can serve as good reminders of the reasons to avoid sexual content at work.

WRITTEN RECOVERY PLANS

For addiction recovery to take place, there must be some bottom-line definition of *sobriety.* For an alcoholic, this definition is clear: Sobriety is the total abstention from the use of alcohol and other mind-altering chemicals. Their sobriety date is when they gave up drugs and alcohol or when they entered into Twelve Step recovery. The recovering alcoholic can then have a clear start date from which to measure the length of his or her sobriety.

A definition of *sobriety* for the recovering cybersex addict can be challenging. Unlike sobriety from the use of substances, sexual sobriety is rarely considered to be complete abstinence from sex. Some recovering people, however, may use complete sexual abstinence (celibacy) for short periods of time. Sexual sobriety is often defined as a written contract between sex addicts and their Twelve Step recovery support group or their therapist/clergy. These contracts, or "sexual recovery plans," involve clearly defined behaviors from which the sex addict has committed to abstain in order to define his or her sobriety. A recovering addict related the following:

> In my head I knew what I needed to change and how I needed to change it. But somehow I always ended up fooling myself and getting back into trouble. In the moment, I would somehow justify why something was OK for me to do, even though I had previously said that it wasn't OK. It wasn't until I wrote

down what I needed to change, and committed to this with another person present, that I found the accountability and clarity to remain sober from my cybersex behaviors.

Creating a Sexual Recovery Plan

The simplest way to create a sexual recovery plan, or sex plan, is to write out a clear set of strictly defined boundaries. In an adaption from the recovery plan suggested by Sex Addicts Anonymous, this is done in the form of three columns that represent the areas needing attention and focus.

1. Column 1—*Actions that I know are shameful, problematic, or hurtful to others and myself.* In this column are listed all of the most concerning sexual or related behaviors that need to be stopped immediately. Avoiding these *behaviors* (not thoughts or fantasies) defines *sobriety.* This definition, in turn, allows the person seeking help to define a sober date, or amount of time elapsed without sexual acting out.

2. Column 2—*Actions or thoughts that I know can lead me toward problem situations.* These include people, places, and experiences that are triggers for acting out. This column is used to define all of the situations that can set up a person to engage in a problematic sexual activity. This is not the sexual activity itself but more a definition of "warning or danger signs."

3. Column 3—*The positive rewards of maintaining sobriety and of refraining from my primary problem activities.* This final column lists examples of all the positive things that are encouraged by not sexually acting out on the computer or otherwise. It offers hope and a vision of the improvements and positive things to come.

Sample Recovery Plan

The following sample recovery plan can be used as a guide in creating your own recovery plan. These definitions should always first be reviewed with at least one other recovering person, therapist, or clergyperson and should not be changed at a later date without thoroughly consulting with one of these individuals.

Column 1—Problematic Actions

- going online to observe any kind of pornography (soft or hard)
- participating in any chat rooms
- reading or downloading any images from newsgroups, porn sites, and so on
- e-mail or instant message communication with anyone who interests me sexually or romantically
- masturbating while online
- looking at any sexually related material in the workplace
- looking at or keeping porn videos or magazines
- contacting prostitutes, escorts, or going to sexual massage parlors
- participating in any type of sexual activity outside of my primary relationship

Column 2—Warning Signs That Sobriety Is in Jeopardy

- getting online when no one else is home
- engaging in any online activity at the office that is not directly work related
- "scanning" the TV channels hoping to catch something exciting or distracting

- not resolving fights with spouse
- lying to myself or others, keeping secrets
- isolating
- working more than forty-five hours a week
- not getting enough sleep or exercise
- skipping my support group meetings or therapy
- feeling overwhelmed, scattered, or guilty
- intense sexual fantasy, excessive sexual objectification of others
- wanting to call or write former sex or dating partners

Column 3—The Positive Rewards of Maintaining Sobriety and Refraining from My Primary Problem Activities

- having more time with loved ones and friends—better relationships
- returning to hobbies and creative activities that bring pleasure
- rediscovering romance with partner
- taking some classes toward a possible new career
- feeling clean and good about self
- having more time for relaxation and fun
- going to movies and ball games
- not needing to worry about sexual disease or getting caught lying
- not having to apologize for being late
- placing greater focus on financial health and stability

The underlying motive for writing a concise sexual recovery plan is to offer the addict an ongoing recovery reminder, even in the face of challenging circumstances. One characteristic of addiction, particularly for cybersex addicts, is difficulty maintaining a clear focus on personal beliefs, values, and goals when faced with situations that potentially involve intensity, arousal, stimulation, and impulsive acting out. The words "Trust me just one more time" and promises like "I really will be good this time" can, at any impulsive moment, go right out the window. Without the clearly written, defined boundaries found in a recovery plan, the sex addict is vulnerable to deciding "in the moment" what action is best for him or her. Unfortunately, most addicts' impulsive decisions do not lead them toward their long-term goals and beliefs. Closely following a sexual recovery plan helps to maintain a clear focus on recovery choices regardless of situation or momentary motive.

Some of the above suggestions on how to create a sexual recovery plan may work for certain people and not for others. Some people will claim that the steps will make life too difficult and get in the way of their work or online priorities. This may be true. Some of the steps in the sample recovery plan may seem trivial, a pain, or just silly. Keep in mind what is at stake and that making real change is the goal. Remember, the recovery process may be a simple one, but it is rarely easily or perfectly carried out.

THE GIFTS OF RECOVERY

The process of making real change and recovering from the effects of cybersex addiction fosters a rediscovery of oneself. For the addict, time formerly spent on obsessive online cruising, flirtation, and "the hunt" may now go into family involvement and work. Creativity previously used for seduction and flirting now is available for hobbies, self-care, and healthy relationship exploration. This self-redefinition allows recovering persons to develop a much clearer understanding of themselves and healthy partnerships.

In recovery, addicts who are not in committed relationships begin to rediscover their self-esteem. They learn how to make healthy choices regarding commitment, dating, and romantic partners. They develop clearer definitions of healthy relationships and develop more meaningful personal boundaries. Recovery for addicts in a partnership brings a deeper understanding of their own and their partner's emotional needs and wants, encouraging them to take more risks toward relationship vulnerability and intimacy. Through recovery, honesty and self-knowledge slowly replace hiding and superficiality. The process can offer a deepening level of maturity and hope for truly loving relationships previously unknown to addicts who have given themselves away online.

SEVEN

Recovery for the Cybersex Addict's Partner

□   □   □

Cybersex addiction affects not only the compulsive user, but also the entire family. Like the cybersex addict, the spouse or partner also needs healing and can benefit from a recovery program.

Suzanne, a thirty-eight-year-old woman, had been married for nine years. Only six months into her marriage, Suzanne accidentally found 25,000 hard-core and child pornography photos on her husband's computer. He claimed he knew nothing about them, but over the next two years similar photos kept appearing on his computer. He finally disclosed that he'd been a sex addict since his early teens and had been a compulsive consumer of Internet pornography for at least six years. Suzanne wrote:

> I was horrified! I could not believe I had married this man! I'd thought I had married "the man of my dreams." After attending counseling and promising that he would not use Internet porn again, he resumed its use. After several months apart, I got back together with him only to find that he had issued yet another false promise. This continued over and over, broken promise after broken promise, until we ended up separating.

Maureen, a thirty-nine-year-old woman, married fourteen years, explained:

> The first time I discovered the porn, I was shocked and hurt. I now see it as part of my codependent behavior. I simply didn't want to believe it happened more than once. I never imagined it was part of a bigger problem. I believed his remorse, yet in the back of my mind, I knew that at some time in the near future he would hurt me again.

Suzanne and Maureen were both about to begin their own journey of healing from the effects of cybersex addiction. Unfortunately, this journey often begins alone because of a belief system that keeps the traveler isolated.

ISOLATION

Feelings of shame, self-blame, and embarrassment about having sexual problems accompany the early days of dealing with a partner's cybersex addiction. These feelings may prevent the spouse from talking with others and asking for help. The resulting isolation only serves to worsen the situation. Covering up for the user is part of this stage.

A forty-six-year-old woman, involved for many years in an abusive marriage, describes why she finally left:

> His behaviors would have been public knowledge had I not shielded and protected him. I kept friends from knowing the truth about my marriage and husband, so that they would continue our friendship. I ended friendships with people who got too close and knew too much. I allowed him to choose my friends and to tape my phone calls. I allowed him to explore three extramarital affairs.

A thirty-three-year-old gay man, in a committed relationship for three years where sex with his cybersex-addicted partner is rare, recounts his experience:

> I do not speak to anyone about this for a couple of reasons: (1) I am too ashamed and embarrassed, and (2) I am aware that people would tell me to "rescue myself" and leave the relationship. Leaving is not what I want to do.

For religious people, the church's teachings may isolate them at a time when they most need support. A forty-one-year-old woman, who identifies herself as a "reborn Christian," wrote of her anguish at her sexually empty marriage and her husband's reliance on computer pornography:

> I withdrew even more and was in emotional turmoil. Nobody knew—not even my closest friends, because I knew the judgment against people who used pornography and what the Christian community would do if they knew. I have been terror-stricken. In some cases, I have sought sympathy. In others, I had retaliatory love affairs with other men. While our home has been a battleground at night, in the morning we kissed and made up. When I finally talked about the issues, some of my friends suggested ending the marriage. I don't believe in that. My husband has sworn great solemn oaths that he was forever done with this online behavior. I believed him when I had no reason to do so. Then, within days, weeks, or months . . . a fresh outburst.

This description offers a sad picture of the consequences of cybersex addiction that spouses or partners must endure. Before they are ready to recognize the unmanageability of their lives and the futility of their efforts to control the addict's behavior, spouses must go through a series of stages that can last weeks, months, or even years. Only at the end of this process can they change their focus from solving the addict's problem to obtaining help for themselves. Based on the experience of many partners of cybersex addicts, we recognize three stages of "pre-recovery."

THE PARTNER'S THREE STAGES OF PRE-RECOVERY

Stage 1: Ignorance/Denial

Although the partner recognizes there is a problem in the relationship, he or she is unaware of the role of cybersex. ("I knew something was wrong the first two years of our marriage, but I could not identify it.") They believe the cybersex addict's denials, explanations, and promises. They tend to ignore their own concerns and may blame themselves for sexual problems in the relationship. When the cybersex addict does not seem interested in marital sex, spouses may try to enhance their own attractiveness by wearing seductive clothing, buying sexual toys, or even attempting to lose weight or have cosmetic surgery. Although their self-esteem is clearly suffering, partners are unlikely to seek help at this point, as they are attempting to "control the problem" themselves.

Late in stage one, the partner may become more suspicious and begin "detective work." However, snooping or other detective behaviors are even more typical of a later stage.

Stage 2: Shock/Discovery

At some point, the partner learns about the true nature of the cybersex activities. The partner may discover this by accident, either while happening upon the addict in the midst of the activity or by finding a cache of pornographic pictures or romantic communications on the computer. Sometimes, the discovery is the result of deliberate investigation.

Discovery of the cybersex activities usually evokes strong feelings of shock, betrayal, anger, pain, hopelessness, confusion, and shame. Addicts often recognize these feelings in their partners and may promise their partners and themselves to give up cybersex. Unfortunately, because the pull of the computer is so strong and its availability in the home and at work is so great, the addict is likely to return to cybersex activities no matter how sincere their initial intentions to quit. Many spouses describe cycles of discoveries, fights, promises made, and later more painful discovery. During stage two, the partner's ignorance and denial abruptly end.

Stage 3: Problem-Solving Attempts

The partner now begins to take action to resolve the problem, which is perceived as the cybersex behaviors. At this stage, the classic behaviors of the sex addict's partner peak—snooping, bargaining, controlling access to the computer, giving ultimatums, asking for full disclosure after every episode, obtaining information for the addict on sex addiction and addiction recovery, and (early in this stage) increasing the frequency and repertory of sexual activities with the addict in hopes of decreasing the addict's desire for cybersex.

Here is the story of a thirty-eight-year-old woman, married eight years:

> The breaking point became his willingness to lie to me to cover his activities and his shame. At some point, I had asked that if he acted out, he tell me right away so that we could work with it. My preference of course was that he come to me when he felt like acting out, but that didn't happen. I could deal with the addiction if it were out in the open, because we

would both begin to gain insights into the why of this complicated issue.

This type of agreement rarely works for long. It only provides a measure of comfort for the partner to know what is going on and offers an illusion of control. Unfortunately, it establishes a parent-child dynamic within the couple relationship. The addict gets resentful and typically ends up lying about his or her behavior.

A forty-one-year-old woman, married twenty-three years, said:

> In the past, I closed off his online accounts, despite feeling like his mother. We have separate screen names, and I have the master screen name and parental controls. I put the controls on and then take them off, feeling guilty to restrict his access. I eventually put them on again because of the behavior.

A forty-seven-year-old woman, married thirty years, admitted:

> I have spied on his e-mail activities. I am computer proficient and he is not. I have deleted his screen name when he could not handle the smorgasbord of women online, as he puts it. I am in charge of the parental controls on AOL. When I gave him his screen name back, I locked him out of chat rooms and had his instant-message access restricted to certain people. This prevents his anonymous cruising.

Partners in stage three believe that additional information will help them manage the situation. This leads to "snooping" or "detective work." Co-addicts who are computer-savvy learn how to trace the addict's activities. In some cases, they may even try to entice the addict by logging into the same chat rooms themselves.

A thirty-five-year-old woman, who six months earlier had discovered her husband's cybersex files on his home computer, wrote:

> I found myself making up screen names to entice him into chatting with me. I wanted to see how far he goes with his cybersex. I have even answered his online personal ads with false information, in response to which he asked for my phone number. When I wasn't with him at night, I would log on to the computer at 2 or 3 A.M. only to find him online in a chat room. I have also checked his computer to see what areas he had visited and what new pictures he had downloaded.

In stage three, when the cybersex activities are exposed, the couple attempts to make an agreement on how to limit the addict's use of the computer. This may consist simply of promises of abstinence or restriction of usage to legitimate needs. Often, the spouse, with the addict's approval or knowledge, assumes control of the access. In addition, filtering software (such as Cyber Patrol or Net Nanny) may be purchased to prevent access to sexually oriented sites, with the nonaddict partner holding the access codes. Keep in mind that these "negative" methods tend to be successful only temporarily if they are not accompanied by "positive" recovery-oriented activities.

At the end of the three stages of pre-recovery, partners of addicts enter true recovery when they accept that they are in crisis and need help. At this point, partners realize that their problem-solving efforts are unsuccessful and the costs of remaining in the status quo become intolerable. Symptoms include depression, isolation, loss of libido, a "dead" marriage, dysfunctional behaviors in some cases (affairs, excessive drinking, violence), and awareness of the effects on the children. In the recovery stage, spouses learn that they are not the cause of the problem and cannot solve it. Once the spouse of the cybersex addict is in therapy and getting help, the marriage or relationship will most likely end unless the cybersex addict also becomes committed to the recovery process.

TAKING STEPS: THE SPOUSE OR PARTNER

Spouses or partners of cybersex addicts can use the following checklist to gauge the health of their own behaviors. If they have experienced three or more of the ten feelings or behaviors, it may be time to seek help.

Partner Checklist

1. attempting to compete with cybersex images—through dress or in sexual behavior
2. participating in sexual activities with the spouse that one is uncomfortable with
3. losing interest in sex with the spouse, because of negative reactions to the spouse's cybersex activities
4. spying on a partner's cybersex activities
5. joining the spouse in cybersex activities in an attempt to control the spouse's cybersex behaviors
6. covering up for a partner's cybersex activities
7. trying to protect children from exposure to the cybersex activity
8. eliciting promises from the spouse to stop cybersex activities
9. insisting on controlling the partner's access to the computer
10. becoming depressed or suicidal in response to the spouse's cybersex activities

When the intimacy of a primary relationship rapidly diminishes and compulsive cybersex is the suspected or known cause, the nonaddicted partner does not have to sit by silently and helplessly watch the adverse consequences of the addiction. Here are some steps partners can take for their own healing:

First Steps

1. Since spouses cannot control their partner's computer behavior or disinterest in relational sex, it is essential for them to reach out for help and support.

2. Shame can keep spouses isolated and sometimes unable to seek counseling or talk with close friends. It is important to confide in at least one friend, relative, or professional who is accepting and nonjudgmental. Contacting an online support group for partners of sex addicts, such as **coanon-approval@MailingList.net,** is another option. This can be done anonymously through an unrecognized screen name while still benefiting from group support.

3. Trust your instincts! When a spouse or partner suddenly becomes unavailable for large blocks of unaccounted time, loses interest in couple sex, appears more distracted and busier than usual without a convincing explanation, becomes more critical of you and less involved with the family—check it out. Evaluate the explanations with a discerning ear. If things don't add up, reserve judgment rather than believe uncritically.

4. Do some "detective" work. Partners often need some real evidence to feel sufficiently empowered to take action.

Next Steps

1. Get support. It doesn't matter whether the cybersex addict admits the behavior and gets help. Being in a relationship with a cybersex addict can result in loss of self-esteem, a sense of betrayal, and the disappearance of trust. Consulting with an understanding counselor and attending a Twelve Step group (live or online) will foster individual and relationship healing.

2. Don't agree to be the keeper of passwords or the supervisor of the addict's time on the computer. Although it is tempting to be actively involved in making sure the addict doesn't "cheat," in the long run assuming a parental role will damage the couple relationship. Ask your partner to consult with a Twelve Step sponsor, counselor, or other recovering person to help manage his or her computer use.

3. Protect children from exposure to cybersex images and sexual activities. If children are being exposed to these experiences, consider a marital separation until the situation changes.

4. Counselors can help set appropriate boundaries for what happens in the home. Some partners may decide that if another episode of real-time online sex takes place in the home, the cybersex addict will have to move out. A caveat: Partners shouldn't give ultimatums unless they are willing to follow through on the consequences.

THE GIFTS OF RECOVERY

For the spouse, recovery can bring a restoration of self-esteem and hope, a validation of long-held feelings about relationship problems, and a restored ability to trust one's own judgment. Spouses in recovery can begin to overcome their shame and self-doubt by joining a community of other people dealing with similar problems. For couples, overcoming deception and rebuilding trust can now begin, culminating in a more emotionally intimate relationship. For the majority of couples whose sexual relationship has significantly deteriorated as a result of the intrusion of cybersex, recovery can bring a healthy and fulfilling sexual relationship. Chapter 8 offers more detailed information about the resources available to cybersex addicts and their partners.

EIGHT

Finding Help

◻ ◻ ◻

THE SIX STAGES OF CHANGE

In their book *Changing for Good*, authors James Prochaska, John Norcross, and Carlos DiClemente describe six stages that people go through in creating life changes.[1] They call these stages (1) precontemplation (resisting change), (2) contemplation (change on the horizon), (3) preparation (getting ready), (4) action (time to move), (5) maintenance (staying there), and (6) termination. These descriptions help clarify the process that cybersex addicts and family members go through in dealing with their problem.

A person in the earliest stage, *precontemplation*, has no intention of changing his or her behavior and typically denies having a problem. Although the person's family, friends, neighbors, doctors, and co-workers can see the problem quite clearly, the precontemplator cannot. As Prochaska and his colleagues note, most precontemplators don't want to change themselves, just the people around them. Denial is characteristic of precontemplators, who blame their problems on factors out of their control, such as genetic makeup, family, society, or "destiny."

Precontemplators deny having a problem even while their family life and job performance suffer.

One important step in beginning to understand the difficult and potentially shameful sexual patterns of cybersex addiction is simply reading this book. The insight and information contained in a book about addictions can help someone move from the early stage of precontemplation into a greater self-awareness. The second stage of change is *contemplation.* In this stage, people acknowledge a problem exists and begin to think seriously about solving it. Recovery from cybersex addiction begins with the all-important acknowledgment that a problem really exists. Once the problem is recognized, then the actual planning toward change can begin.

The third stage of creating change, *preparation*, involves making the final adjustments necessary to prepare for a change in behavior. People in this stage plan carefully, developing a detailed scene for action, and they also begin informing others of their intended change. Smokers, for example, may set a quit date of one week hence, and announce to their families, "I will quit one week from today."

In the *action* stage, people overtly modify their behavior and their surroundings. Recovering cybersex addicts install blocking software, move their computers to a common area of the house, and enlist the help of other recovering people to check in with regarding their computer use. Their recovery program asks them to take a good hard look at themselves by listing their personality traits and behaviors ("defects of character") that require change and read this list to another person. Next, recovering addicts will identify people they have harmed and make sincere amends for the harm caused.

During the *maintenance* stage, recovering addicts work to consolidate the gains they attained during the action and other stages, and struggle to prevent lapses and relapse. Should a lapse or relapse occur, learning from it will further strengthen the lessons learned thus far in the maintenance stage.

The final stage of change described in Prochaska, Norcross, and DiClemente's book is *termination*, a time when a former addiction or problem no longer presents an active temptation or threat. With a lesser continuing effort, people in the termination stage are confident that they can cope with life's problems without relapsing. Because maintaining sobriety from an addiction is an ongoing process, recovering addicts must commit to a lifetime of supportive maintenance.

In recovery from cybersex addiction, support groups, therapists, and online resources can all facilitate movement through the stages of recovery. These resources are described below.

RECOVERY RESOURCES

Peer Support Groups

Self-help groups help addicts to continually grow in their recovery. Fellowships modeled after the Twelve Steps of Alcoholics Anonymous (AA) help millions recover from alcoholism and other addictions, such as pathological gambling, eating disorders, and compulsive sexual behaviors including cybersex addiction. For most of these compulsions and addictions, support groups also exist for spouses and significant others that function like Al-Anon, the group for family and friends of alcoholics.

For many people, one of the hardest initial steps in the healing process is attending their first Twelve Step meeting. It is important to keep in mind that those most successful at long-standing recovery are actively involved in self-help support programs on a regular, long-term basis and use these as a personal safety net for ongoing recovery. Entering a Twelve Step environment can seem confusing or cultish for some, while others feel as if they've come home from the very first visit. People with cybersex addictions often find help in Twelve Step programs such as Sex Addicts Anonymous (SAA), Sexaholics Anonymous (SA), and Sex and Love Addicts Anonymous (SLAA). See appendix 1 for information about contacting these groups.

Basic Tools of Recovery

The Twelve Steps are a deceptively simple program for recovery, originated more than sixty years ago by the founders of AA.

The Twelve Steps of the recovery program are its basic tools. The Steps, modified for recovery from compulsive sexual behaviors, are listed in appendix 1. The first three are belief Steps, the next six are action Steps, and the last three are maintenance Steps. In brief, these Steps are

- recognizing that we cannot solve our problems alone
- believing that an outside force (a Higher Power) can help us
- listing our strengths and faults and describing them to another person
- making restitution for the harm we have caused, whenever possible
- monitoring our thoughts and behavior on an ongoing basis
- continuing to seek spiritual assistance in dealing with our problems
- letting other people who need the same kind of help know about the program

GETTING PROFESSIONAL HELP

Many people who get hooked on online sex seek help from therapists, but not all are successful in finding the right one. Consider the cases of George and Stephen.

George was a fifty-one-year-old married architect with a long-standing addiction to pornography, fantasy, and compulsive masturbation. His cybersex activities cost him time at work, made sex with his wife less intimate and less pleasurable, and distanced him from his family. George admitted to his counselor that he preferred cybersex to sex with his wife and that his behavior was out of control. He explained why he had left his two previous counselors:

> The first therapist I saw did not believe that sex addiction was real. He didn't seem to think there was a problem and suggested that I just had a strong sex drive. This was frustrating, as I know how much suffering the consequences of these behaviors caused me—the cycles of acting out, guilt, shame, and the desire to be free from my compulsions. A second counselor tried to convert me to his religious beliefs. I need a counselor who understands that this is a huge problem for me and can guide me toward recovery.

Stephen was a thirty-seven-year-old single gay man who spent twenty to thirty hours a week online and had isolated himself from friends. His advertising career suffered, he was chronically tired from lack of sleep, and he was on an antidepressant for depression diagnosed by his primary care physician. Stephen recognized he was unavailable for real relationships because of all the time he spent on cybersex. He related, "When I eventually felt that sexual addiction was a serious problem for me and asked my therapist for help with it, he seemed to think my problem was more my self-criticism about my sexual activity than the activity itself." Stephen did not feel understood or validated by his counselor.

The biggest problem among therapists who counsel cybersex users seems to be lack of information about the online experience's power over the cybersex addict. Therapists may lack information about types of online sexual activities and sometimes underestimate their tremendous effect on the user. As a result, the therapist may attempt to make the user more accepting of the activity or attempt to integrate the activity into the user's life by willpower and simple decision making. Therapists need to ask probing questions that will give them a full picture of what the client is doing and how it is affecting his or her life.

Therapists of cybersex addicts make a second error when they fail to make it a priority to stop illegal or self-destructive behaviors. For example, a counselor who was seeing a young man involved in sexual chat and cybersex with underage girls helped him understand the family origins of his behaviors and helped him to no longer feel dirty or ashamed of them, but did not insist that he stop having cybersex with children. The man continued to harm others, as well as to risk arrest. If clients are engaging in high-risk activities, sessions must urgently focus on practical ways to stop the behavior.

A third problem among therapists is failure to consider that the cybersex addict's behavior has consequences for the spouse or partner, consequences that were addressed in chapter 5. It is helpful to involve the addict's significant other in therapy, whether with the same or a different counselor, and to suggest attendance at support groups if such are available.

For addicts who are motivated to change their behavior, a knowledgeable therapist or counselor can help them successfully adapt to that change. Initial topics to be discussed in counseling include the following: (1) understanding how the addictive behavior enables the person to cope, (2) acknowledging the costs of using that particular behavior to reach the desired goal, (3) finding alternative means of tolerating difficult circumstances or feelings, and (4) understanding how the person came to use the particular behavior.

When the behavior harms another person, such as the addict's spouse or significant other, that person may be brought into counseling as well. The couple may then negotiate ways to get past the pain and difficulties caused by the behavior and develop more productive and positive ways of relating.

Choosing a Good Therapist

Cybersex addiction is such a new phenomenon that few therapists are familiar with it. In fact, although twenty years have elapsed since the publication of Dr. Patrick Carnes's groundbreaking book, *Out of the Shadows: Understanding Sexual Addiction,* many therapists are unfamiliar with treating any type of compulsive sexual behavior. For this reason, it is important to find a knowledgeable counselor or therapist.

Because there are so many different types of helping professionals, selecting the right one can be confusing. The choices include a psychiatrist, Ph.D.-level psychologist, addiction medicine doctor, sex therapist, master's-level counselor, social worker, addiction counselor, or pastoral counselor. Instead of focusing on the professional's academic degree, look for someone with training in and knowledge of compulsive sexual behaviors. A background in the addiction field is particularly helpful.

Begin by asking others for names of therapists who specialize in dealing with addictive disorders in general and with cybersex addiction, sex addiction, or compulsive sexual behaviors. People who already attend a Twelve Step meeting because of a cybersex addiction are often helpful in recommending therapists or counselors. Another excellent resource is the National Council on Sexual Addiction and Compulsivity Web site: **www.ncsac.org,** which maintains a list of counselors knowledgeable about sex addiction, arranged by state. Therapists who have expertise in compulsive sexual behaviors are the professionals most likely to know about cybersex addiction. An addiction treatment facility could provide names of knowledgeable therapists in the caller's community. Since addiction treatment programs depend on referrals from therapists, they are often knowledgeable about their professional practices.

Many larger companies and some unions offer their workers access to an employee assistance program (EAP). EAP counselors often have addiction training, though they may not be knowledgeable about compulsive sexual behaviors.

Cybersex addicts who have health insurance need to check their coverage to see what diagnoses are covered and what therapists they can use. Be aware that many plans do not cover treatment for sexual concerns. However, people suffering from a cybersex addiction frequently experience anxiety, depression, marital problems, or situational stress, and can request a referral to a mental health specialist to help with these problems. If the health plan does not cover payment for any therapist knowledgeable about compulsive sexual disorders, paying out of pocket is an option.

After locating a professional in the field, prospective clients should then make an appointment to get acquainted. Ask about the professional's policy regarding billing for this consultation. Some therapists schedule the usual fifty-minute session and bill at their usual rate; others require a lengthy assessment session; still others provide a free consultation. Receiving therapy from the right therapist who is a good fit and who knows how to deal with addictive behaviors, even if it means paying out-of-pocket fees, is money well spent.

An initial consultation with a therapist provides an opportunity to ask questions to determine whether the therapist is a good match for you. This meeting does not, however, commit you to continue therapy with that person. It may take several meetings with the therapist to decide whether this professional can meet your needs.

Questions to Ask a Prospective Therapist

To determine whether a therapist is able to handle cybersex addiction issues, evaluate the therapist's experience, family orientation, and beliefs about secrecy and disclosure of sexual secrets, as well as your comfort level with that therapist.

Experience

Like addiction to alcohol, cybersex addiction is best addressed through addiction treatment. Ask prospective therapists:

1. What is your experience with cybersex addiction, with compulsive sexual behaviors in general, and with other addictions?
2. Do you recommend that your clients attend Twelve Step meetings?
3. Are you familiar with the concepts taught in Alcoholics Anonymous and its offshoots?
4. If you are not familiar with the Twelve Step model, are you supportive of a client's involvement with Twelve Step meetings, and are you willing to learn about the value of Twelve Step meetings?

Family Orientation

Some therapists focus entirely on their individual clients and do not address the effects of the client's behavior on or needs of the client's family members. Cybersex addiction, like other addictive and compulsive disorders, affects the addict's spouse, loved ones, and children. It is desirable to choose a therapist who looks at all aspects of cybersex addiction, including the consequences to the family. Here are some questions to ask prospective family therapists:

1. Do you treat only addicts, or do you also treat family members for the consequences of the addiction?
2. Do you work as a part of a team with other therapists to help a family or couple, if needed?
3. If you treat family members, is the primary goal of treatment to help the addict's recovery, or do you consider family members clients in their own right?
4. If a spouse complains about the cybersex addict's use of pornography and/or involvement with real-time on-line sex partners, do you perceive these activities to be trivial compared with "real" affairs or adultery, or do you understand the damage that these behaviors can inflict on a relationship?

It may take considerable discussion or more than one time together for the client to have a clear picture of the therapist's perspective.

Secrecy and Disclosure

In recovery from any addiction, addicts are often told, "You are as sick as your secrets." Just as keeping secrets is a part of the inner workings of any active addiction, honesty is a crucial element in recovery from all addictive disorders. What is often unclear to people entering recovery is how much to reveal and what issues are best kept a secret. Counselors have different approaches to this difficult problem. Consider the following situations:

Leonard and Laura

Leonard, a thirty-six-year-old accountant, came to see Dr. Jones for marriage counseling at the urging of his wife, Laura, who became extremely upset after finding a stash of pornographic pictures on their home computer as well as numerous erotic e-mail exchanges from other women. Before seeing them as a couple, Dr. Jones saw Leonard and Laura individually and gathered a sexual history from each. Leonard privately admitted to the therapist that he'd met several of the online women in person and had had sex with them. He asked her not to reveal this information to his wife, who believed that he had engaged in online sex only. Leonard assured Dr. Jones that he was not currently involved with any of the women, so there was no need for Laura to know about his past. He said he was attending a Twelve Step program for sex addicts, had installed blocking software on the home computer and moved it to the family den, and felt he had a good handle on his previous behavior.

In her individual session with Dr. Jones, Laura said she felt betrayed by and distrustful of her husband, who had lied to her about his cybersex involvement (he'd told her he was working late at the home computer on an accounting project). Laura also said that she was angry that Leonard said she was making a mountain out of a molehill and did not take her concerns seriously enough.

Dr. Jones saw Leonard and Laura for six sessions. Meetings focused on improving communication between the two, doing caring gestures for each other, and arranging for some fun one-on-one activities away from the children. The couple was making good progress in therapy, but one day, while driving to Dr. Jones's office, where she was going to meet Leonard, Laura discovered a strange earring in Leonard's jacket, which had been lying on the back seat of the car. Walking into the therapy session, she immediately confronted Leonard, who promptly owned up his past affairs. He also told Laura that he'd informed Dr. Jones about this at the onset of therapy.

Laura's reaction was anger not only at Leonard, but also at Dr. Jones, who had colluded with Leonard in the dishonesty. Laura felt she'd been betrayed by *two* people whom she had trusted and that the therapy sessions had been a waste of time because they had not addressed what in retrospect was the most important single issue in the marriage—the affairs and the dishonesty around them. She was further enraged in discovering that her husband had practiced unprotected sex with several of these women, endangering her own health! Yet Dr. Jones had not asked Leonard about this, and Leonard had not brought this information to her. Furious and hurt, Laura declined to continue in couples therapy with Dr. Jones. She and Leonard separated soon thereafter.

Mitch and Margaret

Mitch, a forty-three-year-old computer programmer, came to see Mr. Adams for marriage counseling at the insistence of his wife, Margaret. She was very distressed after learning that her husband had been downloading pornographic images from the Internet and engaging in cybersex with several other women online. Before counseling them as a couple, Mr. Adams met with Mitch and Margaret separately and obtained a sexual history from each. Like Leonard in the previous story, Mitch admitted to the therapist that he'd met several of the online women in person and had had sex with them. He requested that Mr. Adams keep this information from Margaret, who believed that her husband's indiscretions had been limited to online sex. Mitch assured Mr. Adams that he was no longer involved with any of the women, was attending Twelve Step meetings, and had a good handle on his previous behavior.

Mr. Adams refused to counsel the couple if Mitch didn't reveal his secret to Margaret, since it was a critical part of the couple's problems. He explained to Mitch that he could not offer effective marriage therapy if such important issues were not discussed during sessions. He also noted that he could not have an honest therapeutic relationship with Margaret if he was withholding significant information from her. Mr. Adams reminded Mitch that honesty is a key ingredient in addiction recovery and that an important goal of therapy after infidelity is for the couple to rebuild trust in each other.

Mitch admitted he was afraid that Margaret would leave him if she knew the truth. After validating that this is a very common fear, Mr. Adams explained that although many partners threaten to leave after learning of an affair, far fewer actually do so. Mr. Adams offered to work with Mitch individually for up to three sessions to figure out how to best disclose the affairs to Margaret. He recommended that the disclosure take place during a joint therapy session, so they could all then work together to resolve the resulting feelings. Mr. Adams advised Mitch that if, after the three sessions, he was still not ready to come clean with Margaret, then Mr. Adams would continue doing individual work with Mitch, but would not provide marriage counseling with the couple.

After preparing himself in two individual sessions with Mr. Smith, Mitch did tell Margaret about his affairs during a joint therapy session. Mitch told Margaret that he was committed to the marriage and wanted to work things out, no matter what it took to do so. Mr. Adams offered to Margaret the option of meeting with another counselor to work through her distress and anger over Mitch's affairs, but she instead chose to meet a few times with Mr. Adams for individual sessions. A stormy period in the couple's marriage resulted, but their sessions continued with Mr. Adams. Their therapy sessions for the next few months focused on rebuilding trust, building safety into the relationship, and getting beyond the hurts of the past.

Dr. Jones and Mr. Adams chose very different approaches in dealing with secret affairs within the context of couple counseling. Although some therapists still adopt the approach demonstrated by Dr. Jones, many more recognize that colluding with one partner in keeping such a secret is very likely to adversely affect the therapy process. Facilitating disclosure as part of the couples' therapy is a more effective approach, in particular with families who are working on recovering from addiction.[2]

Active addiction usually involves secrets. Spouses and partners may be unaware that the compulsive cybersex user has had sexual encounters with people both online and offline. When interviewing therapists, it is essential to ask how they deal with secrets. The following questions might serve as a guide:

1. What is your position on the cybersex user keeping secrets about past and present sexual behaviors?
2. Are you comfortable knowing about such affairs or encounters and not disclosing this information to the spouse?
3. What is your position about the disclosure of information to the couple's children and/or family members about the addiction?

These questions are particularly relevant if both partners will be working with the same therapist.

Getting Help in Nonurban Areas

Urban areas offer a variety of therapists to choose from and daily self-help meetings of all types. People living in rural areas, on the other hand, may have limited access to meetings. Yet this doesn't mean that help is unavailable to those living in less-populated areas. Some useful resources follow:

- Several Twelve Step sexual recovery programs have online meetings and offer long-distance peers and sponsors by phone and/or e-mail communication. Many recovering people participate in regular weekly recovery chats online, while gaining strength and support from around the world. People without Internet access can connect to others by phone. Twelve Step programs also regularly publish newsletters and have other reading materials (available through the mail or online). Twelve Step programs also hold annual conventions in different parts of the United States. This is a great opportunity to connect with others in recovery.
- Some therapists are willing to do counsel clients via the telephone or through e-mail exchanges. You can find professionals trained in cybersex and sexual addiction recovery in the geographic listing at the National Council on Sexual Addiction and Compulsivity's Web site **www.ncsac.org.**
- There are also books and Web sites devoted to sex addiction recovery (of which cybersex is a part). These books and materials are available through online bookstores, libraries, and local bookstores. A list of suggested reading can be found in appendix 1.

HELP FOR THERAPISTS

Because cybersex activities are solitary and often secretive, therapists who do not ask the right questions may miss the diagnosis. Important questions to ask are listed in the Cybersex Addiction Checklist and the Male Sexual Addiction Screening Test (G-SASF) in appendix 1. In our survey of spouses and partners of cybersex addicts, several reported unproductive experiences with professionals. Some counselors had never heard of sexual addiction or compulsivity and concluded that the problem was insufficient sex for the cybersex user. Their solution was for the partner to initiate sex more frequently. Others were so committed to being nonjudgmental that they missed the big picture.

A twenty-nine-year-old woman, newly married, confided:

> It scared me that my fiancé went to Internet sites to see young girls [fourteen years old and older]. Before we were married, I talked with my pastor about it, and he suspected it was just curiosity. He concluded that once we were married, my husband's curiosity would be filled by me. We are now married, and he has continued his acting out. He has lied to me so much that I am afraid of what could happen if we have children and one is a girl.

Clients' complaints about their spouses' cybersex use may simply reflect their own discomfort with pornography, or it may be a sign of cybersex addiction. Each of these requires a different treatment approach. When sexual compulsivity is present, potential mistakes by the uninformed therapist include the following:

1. underestimating the adverse consequences of the behavior

2. diagnosing the couple's problem as either poor communication, the partner's frigidity, or a need by the partner for greater acceptance of the Internet user's activities

3. diagnosing the addict's problem as a lack of sexual drive or interest, whereas the cybersex addict is actually very sexually active (with the computer, not the spouse)

4. recommending prematurely that the cybersex user limit the time devoted to cybersex activities to some predetermined number of hours, or to have the partner join in the addict's cybersex activities

The Importance of Gathering Information

The first step for the counselor is to gather information, preferably from both partners, separately and together, by asking very specific questions, such as the following:

1. What is a typical day in the life of each partner?
2. Are there large chunks of either partner's time that are unaccounted for?
3. Have there been changes in the couple's sexual relationship?
4. Have there been changes in the amount of time the family spends together?
5. Have there been changes in the time spent with children?
6. Is there evidence of cybersex involvement?
7. Is there a history of other compulsive sexual behaviors?

Counselors should ask about each partner's beliefs and activities regarding sex, pornography, and masturbation. A *thorough* sexual history from both partners and a history of their sexual relationship with each other should be obtained.

Treating Cybersex Addiction: Addict and Partner

If cybersex addiction is indeed present, the basic treatment principles are the same as with any form of sexual addiction. Initially, the addict needs help to

- break through the denial that a problem exists
- recognize the impact of the behaviors on the partner and family
- stop the behaviors and associated lying
- stop blaming the partner
- learn problem-solving techniques
- develop strategies for dealing with sexual urges (see chapter 6, pages 113–119, for specific strategies for computer use)

As with other addictions, partners of cybersex addicts benefit from ongoing counseling. Partners need validation that a problem really does exist and that cybersex addiction can be just as damaging to relationships as traditional sexual affairs. They need to feel "heard" by the counselor and encouraged to state their needs. Other early goals are to help spouses accept that they did not cause, cannot control, and cannot cure the problem. It is important for partners to overcome the false belief that by acquiring enough information, they can somehow control the situation. They need to realize that one person cannot control another's behavior for long. Partners need to stop trying to fix the other person and begin focusing on themselves. Healing a damaged self-esteem and learning to pay attention to one's own needs and desires are important. Education about appropriate boundaries is essential, especially regarding the presence of the home computer and conditions for its use.

For the spouse or significant other, the physical presence of the computer itself gives the problem an immediacy and visibility often absent in other addictions that can be better hidden. It is not generally useful to have the partner be the "keeper" of the computer or to control the cybersex addict's use of it. This is better left to the addict's therapist or sponsor. Like the cybersex addict, the partner can be greatly helped and supported by a Twelve Step program such as S-Anon, Codependents of Sex Addicts (COSA), or Al-Anon. For more information on these programs, see appendix 1.

MANAGING RELAPSE

Juan's Story

Before getting into trouble again, I had been actively working to manage my cybersex problem for several months. Before starting recovery, I spent up to five hours nightly in sexual chats and cruising porn sites. During my first few months of recovery, I was involved in some therapy, attended weekly Twelve Step meetings, and regularly worked on learning about the problem. I began to regard my past behavior as a reflection of a difficult time in my life that was now ending.

When I passed the five-month mark in recovery, I guess I gradually became less serious about some earlier commitments, such as not going online when at home alone or after hours at the office. I never found the time to install the blocking software I bought to keep me out of inappropriate sites. One Saturday when the family was out, I thought, "I should really just relax today and take some time for me. I deserve it." So I slept in instead of going to my regular Saturday support group meeting. That morning it occurred to me that I could view my stock portfolio service online. After observing the stocks, I began to check out other sites of interest, such as sports, news, and travel. I was impressed with myself at how well I was handling the online activity.

I continued to view one of the sports sites until encountering a link to "check out the latest swimsuit models live." Without a second thought, I just clicked the link, saying, "I'll just look at a few photos. After all, bathing suits aren't porn." A few photos soon led to more bathing suit photos and eventually to more explicit sites. After spending two and a half hours that day online, viewing porn and masturbating, I realized that I really didn't have any control over my behavior. Unless I followed the plan that had been suggested to me—to the letter—I wasn't going to really get well.

Juan's story demonstrates how cybersex addicts can relapse by thinking they are cured. Juan didn't overtly start out looking for sex, though he now recalls feeling mildly excited about being home alone and also feeling entitled to it. He thought, I deserve to be able to have this time to myself to look at this. I have been working so hard. It's a good reward. More important, Juan's story helps outline some important signs of impending relapse.

Key Warning Signs of Relapse

- minimizing the return to problematic situations ("Oh, these sites aren't nearly as graphic as the ones I used to view. Look, I am not even downloading the images.")
- lying to self and others
- skipping or devaluing feedback from others ("I don't need that support group, therapy, or outreach phone call anymore. I'm doing fine on my own.")
- overconfidence ("This has gone really well for a few months; maybe I have the problem licked.")

- isolation
- blaming others ("If she just would put the kids to bed earlier and give me some time to myself, I wouldn't be online as much.")
- feeling victimized by not having complete online freedom ("Others get to be online and look at whatever they want. Why can't I sometimes look at attractive women?")
- ignoring previously agreed upon guidelines
- feeling entitled to return to some of the formerly problematic behaviors ("Look how hard I have been working in the office and at home, not to mention my recovery. What difference would it make if I just looked at a little porn here and there? I deserve a break.")
- making excuses and setting up problematic situations ("I have got to get this report done. If I stay late at the office after everyone leaves, what's the big deal?")

Avoiding Relapse

In Twelve Step programs, recovering people are awarded medallions representing their days, months, or years of continuous sobriety. A relapse causes the clock to be set back to zero. No wonder some addicts who relapse get discouraged, believing that they have to start from scratch again. In reality, relapses are often a painful but common feature of addictive disorders. They are not a sign of weak character or abject failure. A relapse indicates that a person's recovery program has some weak links. Reviewing the steps that led to the relapse helps the addict identify the weak links and set in place new elements that will strengthen the recovery program and help prevent additional relapses.

One message is clear: Cybersex recovery cannot be achieved

in isolation—either alone or as a couple. People who are actively involved in an addiction and those deeply and directly affected by it need the support, direction, and clarity of others who understand both the problem and the paths to a solution. Outreach to a Twelve Step program, other support group, or a professional counselor is important. It is not an indication of shame or weakness on the part of the person seeking help. Rather, reaching out demonstrates courage and a willingness to admit there is a problem that requires the support and understanding of others.

NINE

On the Road to Recovery

▣　▣　▣

People who are lost in the labyrinth of the cybersex world sometimes wonder if they will ever find their way out. Even when they see clearly that their current path is destructive to themselves and others, the prospect of change may seem overwhelming. This chapter will describe some practical ways for negotiating the journey.

Recovering from any addiction requires more than simply stopping the addictive behavior. It's a recovery of one's sense of self, life, and healthy pleasure. Although the "do's" of the recovery process reviewed in chapter 8 are the tools that bring the addict to a change in behavior, there is more that must be done to effect long-term change. Change occurs through a commitment to self-care and acknowledging that this process goes far beyond going to therapy or Twelve Step meetings. Consider John's story.

STRUGGLING WITH RECOVERY

John, a forty-seven-year-old married sales executive, was struggling with his recovery process. For many years he was involved in phone sex and porn with compulsive masturbation. He had "graduated" in recent years to pay-per-view online porn memberships and to downloading hundreds of porn photos from newsgroups. Committed to ending these behaviors, John had been attending Twelve Step sex addiction meetings for nearly a year and had spent twice that time in regular weekly therapy. He had been prescribed Prozac for depression, which significantly improved his mood. He had not engaged in cybersex for more than ten months, yet he continued to struggle almost daily with the desire to return to his porn use. A review of John's therapy session revealed why:

John: I don't understand it. I am working so hard in every area of my recovery. I am being absolutely honest with my wife; I am attending several Twelve Step meetings a week and two kinds of therapy. I am writing in my journal daily and working as hard as I can. Every spare moment that doesn't go into work and family goes into my recovery. Yet, I still find myself so obsessed with wanting to act out sexually.

Therapist: It sounds as if you are really working hard in every area of your life. But something still feels like it is missing.

John: Yes, I do feel like something is missing; it must be. Otherwise I wouldn't be so obsessive and distracted.

Therapist: Well John, let's discuss this a bit. What are you doing to take care of yourself?

John: I told you. I am going to meetings and therapy, I write every day . . . spend time with my kids.

Therapist: Yes, John, that is all super for you and the family, but what are you doing for fun?

John: Fun? Well, it's not like I have time for play right now, Doc. I barely have time to undress before bed. I have some serious catching up to do on my work and family life.

Therapist: I guess we are beginning to see the problem here, John.

John: What do you mean?

Therapist: Well, recovery isn't just about dedicating yourself to the work. Recovery is a process of finding yourself, enjoying your life, and making it work. Your life sounds like it is nothing but work—you have replaced the intensity of your sexual acting-out behavior with filling every minute with work. How does that help you make peace with yourself? Tell me, John, how many hours a week are you working in the office?

John: About fifty to sixty hours, depending on the week. Usually I work most of Saturday to catch up.

Therapist: Mmm . . . I thought the work week was supposed to be forty hours or so.

John: Maybe for some people, but I have responsibilities, and I have to respond to the needs of everyone around me to keep driving the business. That is not a forty-hour-a-week job.

Therapist: Oh, I see. And what about your needs, John? Your need for play, for relaxation, and for a quiet spiritual life? Who is going to take responsibility for those? You see, if you don't take care of yourself in a nurturing way, rather than a punishing, driven way, you will end up meeting those needs through sex and pornography. You will find yourself back where you started.

In this scenario, the therapist is able to show John that what's really missing from his recovery is a commitment to take care of himself, not just through therapy, meetings, writing, and meeting everyone else's needs, but by finding *healthy* pleasures and satisfaction in his daily existence. It is essential that recovering people (both addicts and spouses) begin to explore how they can find enjoyment and satisfaction in their daily lives. When dealing with pain or loss, it is important to take time for relaxation, self-reflection, and fun.

THE IMPORTANCE OF SELF-NURTURING

People with addictive and co-addictive problems often have difficulty taking time out just for themselves or even thinking that they should. Addicts' partners and spouses (co-addicts) often focus on making sure that everyone around them has their wants and needs met, but place themselves last. Addicts, in contrast, tend to be intensity focused. Often unable to find peace and quiet within, cybersex addicts seek intense external events and experiences to distract themselves. When addicts and their partners enter the recovery phase, spouses may still find themselves focused on others—specifically, what the addict needs to do to get better—rather than on how they can nurture themselves. Sex addicts are also unaccustomed to nurturing themselves; in the past they used sexualized experiences to distract themselves from feelings of emptiness and inner discomfort that can only be filled through self-care. The concepts of "doing nothing" for a day or finding pleasure in a hobby are often foreign ideas.

Nurturing Tasks for the Individual—Addicts and Partners (Co-Addicts):

The following are suggestions on how to find time for self-nurturing in the midst of a busy life. These concerns are just as critical to the process of creating change—for individuals and couples—as the more "serious" components.

Attend to Nonsexual Friendships

When cybersex addicts are actively addicted, they usually have little going on in their personal lives beyond the addictive behaviors. Absorption in their online fantasy life prevents them from being aware of any loneliness or isolation they might otherwise feel. Even if they are active socially and appear to be close to others, it is rare for addicts to admit the all-consuming nature of their sexual behaviors. Their spouses often find themselves alone, even when the addict is physically present. Those who know about the cybersex addict's activities often feel too embarrassed to talk about it with friends and other supportive people, and instead remain isolated and unhappy.

Isolation is a hallmark of addiction. People in recovery, whether addict or partner, need others in addition to spouses or family members with whom they can discuss their painful challenges and losses. This fellowship—often encouraged through participation in Twelve Step recovery programs, but also obtained by reconnecting with old friends—makes a significant difference in each person's growth. Even though it may be embarrassing at first to discuss such concerns, the support and acceptance that comes with reaching out to a safe person can far outweigh any adverse consequences.

Meditate

Long encouraged by religious groups and Twelve Step programs, regular meditation can create more peace and calm within. Finding ways to create such calm and peace helps the addict avoid the distraction of intensity and arousal. Taking classes or finding a good book about meditation is the easiest way to start. Suggested books include *Mindfulness in Plain English* by Venerable Henepola Gunaratana (Wisdom Publications); *Wherever You Go, There You Are* by Jon Kabat-Zinn (Hyperion); and *Answers in the Heart: Daily Meditations for Men and Women Recovering from Sex Addiction* (Hazelden).

Exercise

In their intense pursuit of gratification from sex or drugs, addicts usually neglect their bodies. This is why addiction treatment programs typically include physical fitness regimens as one element of the recovery plan. Achieving balance in life means paying attention to one's physical fitness as well as emotional and spiritual health. Aside from all the benefits of physical self-care and weight loss, exercising induces many of the same neurochemical changes in the brain that are produced by intensity-based addictions such as online sexual acting out—only in a much healthier fashion. Even the simplest exercise routine (like daily walking), used consistently and in a committed fashion, will significantly increase feelings of serenity, peace, and self-care.

Avoid the "Overwhelm"

Active addicts have a very unbalanced life. They pay too much attention to the addiction and not enough to friends, romantic partners, family, children, or the demands of work. Often, addicts and partners spend their lives frantically putting out fires and playing catch-up to commitments that have been ignored at work and at home. Much of the time, life is lived "in overwhelm." When the addict feels too overwhelmed, the handiest solution is more of the addictive substance or behavior.

In recovery, the solution to overwhelm is to set appropriate priorities and boundaries for work commitments, self-care, and personal relationships. Establishing a plan for the maximum number of hours to be worked per week and commitments to family, friends, and self-care time are useful toward attaining and maintaining balance in one's life and a sense of control.

Spend Time in Nature

Addicts and partners (co-addicts) often feel very isolated and alone. One of the goals of a Twelve Step fellowship is to provide the addict with a community. Another powerful way of realizing that we are not alone, but rather a part of a vast universe, is to spend some time in nature. Outdoors in nature, the interconnectedness of life is realized—a visit to Mount Saint Helens in the Northwest United States makes clear the devastation that a brief volcanic eruption can have upon hundreds of square miles for decades to come. A trip to the Grand Canyon in Arizona shows how over time a river can carve a huge rift in solid rock. A walk in the woods illustrates how birds depend on trees to build their nests, on worms to feed their offspring, on their partner to incubate their eggs. Interdependence, not isolation, is the rule of nature—a good one for recovering people to remember.

Own a Pet

Medical studies have shown that older people who have pets are happier and healthier than people who don't share their lives with animals. When asked to give an example of unconditional love, most people immediately think of the love of a dog for its owner. Pets can immeasurably enhance the life of people. Having a dog or cat to greet you at the door when you come home from work, keep you company when reading or watching TV, or entice you out of the house for a walk can help keep "alone" from becoming "lonely." Moreover, caring for the physical and emotional needs of another living being, whether human or animal, can give a different focus to life besides just worrying about oneself.

Spend Time on Hobbies, Sports, Games, and "Having Fun"

In recovery, it's easy to become focused solely on Twelve Step meetings, therapy sessions, spending quality time with the kids, and other goal-oriented activities neglected during the active addiction. Recreation is often avoided. When life becomes busy and complex, taking time out for travel, hobbies, sports, and other "nonproductive" activities may seem silly. However, it's essential to recharge your battery. It provides the self-nurturing that makes one ready to go out again and succeed at work, relationships, and other aspects of life. The key to a productive and psychologically healthy life is to have balance, and recreation is an important part of this.

Practice Healthy Dating

Recovering from sexual compulsivity does not mean avoiding dating, romance, or healthy sexual expression. For the recovering single cybersex addict, it is important over time to introduce some plan for healthy dating and romance. *Healthy* means following a carefully thought-out action plan that includes boundaries about what period of time dating must take place before having sex. A clear understanding on how to meet partners that encourage healing rather than addiction is needed. Therapy and supportive others help negotiate this sometimes-tricky path.

Create a "Home" at Home

Often, active addicts are too busy with their addiction to focus on making their home a warm and welcoming environment.

Ignoring their emotional or "inner" selves, they readily ignore their "outsides" as well. They do not take the time to nurture a garden, paint a guest room, buy flowers weekly, or arrange the furniture. The simple acts of improving one's home and taking daily or weekly steps to maintain it reflect an important commitment to self-care. It provides a reminder of the ongoing positive change that ending an addiction can bring.

Nuturing Tasks for the Couple

Make Dates for Time Together

In our busy lives it's easy to allow time to slip away without really making time for our partnerships. The expected distractions of work, family, kids, recovery work, friends, and so on can easily take precedence for couples over spending time together alone. Yet studies have proven the need for couples to make the time to be together. This is especially true for recovering couples who carry the burden of past problems and distance. Although making advance preparations seems unromantic, it is essential that couples *plan* times to spend together. The goal is to make actual dates—unbreakable except in an emergency—for the couple to spend time together in play and relaxation. Whether a trip to the beach or an evening on the town, couples need time away from stress and distraction for growth and healing.

Practice Listening/Empathy

Knowing how to listen to one another and make time for sharing is an effective tool for helping couples grow closer. One way to develop this skill is to set aside several specific times each week for listening to each other. This thirty-minute exercise is best carried out when the distractions of the day have ended and there are a few quiet moments. The couple sit facing each other. Each partner has ten minutes of uninterrupted time to say whatever he or she wants to the other person. This can be about the day, feelings, work, and family—anything the person wants to say. The last ten minutes of the session is for both to discuss what they have heard and how they feel about it. This simple exercise should be carried out two to three times each week. It goes a long way toward helping couples establish intimacy and closeness.

Find Shared Activities

Couples in recovery need to find time for activities that stimulate and interest one another. Hiking, gardening, playing sports, going to museums or antique stores are all examples of potentially relationship-growing activities. Experiences that take the couple and/or family out of their daily routine or simply out of the house for fun create a bonding and shared intimacy that no therapy session can offer.

Practice Nonsexual Touch and Holding

Many patients who have issues with sexuality and cybersex grew up in homes where they experienced very little touch and witnessed little or innappropriate physical intimacy. Couples need to work on building physical closeness that is not focused on sex. Hand-holding, hugs, cuddling, bathing together, massages, shoulder rubs, and kisses all offer warmth and validation that cannot be achieved through words alone. Children raised by parents who are physically affectionate with each other also greatly benefit from the healthy closeness and reassurance that this brings.

Introduce Romance

As the couple moves toward forgiveness and healing, romantic interactions work to develop intimacy—not sex per se, but rather the actions people take at the beginning of a relationship to make each other feel loved and appreciated. Notes, cards, flowers, unexpected compliments, surprise gifts, and future plans all work to reestablish the romance. These activities are better carried out in the later stages of recovery than in the early stages. The addict should not use them in an attempt to gain quick forgiveness from the partner. Rather, in a partnership where both people have been working toward establishing trust, romantic interactions help bring closeness and warmth back into the relationship.

REBUILDING TRUST WITH SELF AND IN A PARTNERSHIP

Most cybersex addicts have lied, covered up, manipulated, and hidden their secret lives from those close to them. No wonder loved ones feel betrayed and violated, finding trust difficult—if not impossible. Even when former cybersex addicts follow a strict recovery program, studies have shown that it often takes a year or two before their partners stop doubting their activities. Unfortunately, some partners never regain confidence in the addict. Clearly, the healing process for a relationship involves many steps toward rebuilding trust and gaining healthy intimacy.

Following are steps that couples can take to help repair a damaged relationship. Several steps can help to rebuild trust. Steps for *addicts* include

- practicing rigorous honesty daily with self and others in both small and larger issues
- developing empathy for the pain the partner and other loved ones have experienced

- allowing the partner time to rebuild trust by letting him or her feel anger and mistrust without expecting an immediate "all is forgiven"
- spending time with a partner in activities that the partner enjoys (This might mean going to a movie the partner particularly wants to see, an art show, or a baseball game. The addict's willingness to partake in such an activity demonstrates to the partner that his or her interests are important.)
- establishing and maintaining a stable and consistent plan for self-care
- committing to and maintaining a clear plan for recovery

Steps for *partners* include

- committing to their own personal recovery program
- working on being less judgmental and critical by showing a greater willingness to acknowledge their part in the couple's problems
- becoming willing *over time* to grow beyond anger and betrayal, finding a path toward trust

Steps for *couples* include

- committing to an active recovery program as a couple (couples therapy, Twelve Step couples support groups such as Recovering Couples Anonymous, weekend retreats and workshops)
- spending time together to develop closeness and intimacy (going out on dates, having listening sessions, exercising together, and so on)

Rigorous Honesty

The best antidote for a past life of secrecy and dishonesty is a present life of rigorous honesty in all areas, small and large. It takes many days, weeks, and months of consistency to overcome the distrust that cybersex addicts have earned by their past behavior. If the cybersex addict is going to be home late, it helps to phone the partner and explain why. If he or she has agreed to pick up some milk on the way home but forgets, it is better to admit this memory lapse than to make up some excuse. If the addict needs to use the computer at home, it is better to locate it in a high-traffic area of the home than to keep it behind a closed door while expecting the partner to believe that nothing inappropriate is going on.

Nick, a forty-one-year-old accountant, had affairs both online and offline. His wife, Nancy, was devastated when she first learned about the repeated betrayals. She felt completely blindsided, having had no inkling that the time missing from his schedule had been spent having sex with other women on the computer and offline. Nick talked about how Nancy gradually came to trust him again:

> It's been a gradual process. I realized I had to be completely honest, in small things as well as large. I made sure to be home when I was supposed to. If I had a change of plans, I would always phone or leave a note. For a long time I kept on that straight and narrow, even if I had to go out of my way. It took about a year until I didn't need to do that anymore. If I was going to be late, I didn't have to rush to a phone to let Nancy know why; she was no longer sitting at home tapping her fingers and wondering where I was if I was five minutes late. As Nancy became more willing to trust her gut feelings, she no longer needed all those reassurances.

Individual Recovery Programs

It is very comforting for the spouse or partner of a cybersex addict to see the addict fully engaged in recovery work—attending self-help meetings, going to a counselor, becoming involved in couples counseling, and putting into action the activities that make it safer for the addict to use the computer (such as moving it in a common area of the home, installing blocking software, putting time limits on its use). Ongoing involvement in such activities helps persuade the spouse that the cybersex addict is sincere about changing his or her life.

Partners also benefit from their own recovery work. Counseling and self-help groups can lead to improved self-esteem and less reactivity on the partner's part. It is also likely to help them become more willing to again risk vulnerability with their spouse. Partners in recovery learn to trust their perceptions and judgment and, therefore, become empowered. Once they rely on their gut feelings to inform them that something is wrong, they are more likely to risk trusting again.

After two years of counseling and Twelve Step work, Nancy is willing to trust Nick again. The reason is not only that he has acknowledged the problem and got help, but also because she trusts herself more. Nancy explains:

> If Nick had another affair, I would leave him. I know that today I would know long before it happened. It wouldn't be like it was before, because I could spot the signs right away, even without any detective work. I'm a different person now, more independent, more sure of myself. Before, I was certain that the kids and I would starve out there. That's what Nick kept telling me then. Now I have enough faith in my Higher Power that He would get me through.

Developing Greater Empathy and Patience, with Less Judgment

Both partners need to develop greater empathy for the other person. Going to couples counseling and attending support group meetings with other couples can help facilitate this process. It is often easier to empathize with someone else's partner than with one's own spouse, whose behaviors may be particularly irritating and provoking. Listening to other couples talk about their problems and their efforts to resolve them often helps people better understand their own partner.

Cybersex addicts in early recovery often experience a real sense of loss at having to give up their addictive behavior. They also feel a great deal of shame about their past behaviors and cover-up attempts. These feelings may be so overwhelming that they cannot relate to the hurt and sense of betrayal their partner feels; they don't stop and consider how it must feel to have your partner choose a fantasy sex partner over you. Listening carefully to one's partner, reversing roles and role-playing the partner in a therapy session, and hearing other people's stories can all facilitate the development of empathy. If partners feel that their pain is understood, they are more likely to believe that the cybersex user will not hurt them again. The addict must be willing to be patient with the partner.

Partners of cybersex addicts are often focused on their own hurt, betrayal, and injury to their self-esteem, and they blame the cybersex user. They fail to see that the addict is experiencing a real loss in giving up the computer sex. They tend to be judgmental and see the addict as the only one with a problem, while they see themselves as innocent victims. This adds to the cybersex addict's feelings of shame and low self-esteem. Counseling, listening carefully to the addict, role-playing the addict in therapy sessions, and listening to other cybersex addicts tell their stories can all help build empathy in the partner and melt away the judgmental thinking.

Jessica, a fifty-year-old critical-care nurse, had a very demanding career. Paul, her husband of twenty-five years, had recently retired and became very interested in surfing the Internet on his new computer. Eleven years earlier, Paul had begun a recovery program for sex addiction after admitting to multiple affairs. His problem behaviors had ceased so many years ago that when Paul began staying up late at the computer, it never occurred to Jessica that he was involved in anything sexual. She noticed that he seemed to lose interest in sex with her, but she told herself this was typical of a long-term marriage. Eventually, he admitted to her that he had begun engaging in cybersex. He was viewing pornography and masturbating, as well as exchanging sexually oriented e-mails with other women.

Jessica was initially furious, but soon realized that some marital issues had predisposed Paul to his relapse. Because she was so preoccupied with her work while he had time on his hands, he felt unneeded and unappreciated. Paul resumed active involvement in a Twelve Step program for sex addiction. He set up guidelines for himself for computer use, such as not using it late at night, and installed blocking software and signed up with a family-oriented Internet service provider.

By attending counseling together and making a commitment to sit and talk each day, going out on weekly dates, spending more time together on weekends, and maintaining their own personal recovery Steps, Jessica and Paul were slowly able to attain a new level of intimacy.

Learning to Trust Oneself

Trusting oneself involves the ability to take in cues from the outside world, monitor one's visceral as well as intellectual responses to the cues, and formulate an appropriate response. People who are primarily focused on an addiction are not free to assess and respond to outside cues. Their inner life has already been hijacked by the preoccupation and obsession that is characteristic of addictive disorders. This is why addicts are often unaware of the damage they have caused and the hurt they have inflicted on others. We call this feature of addiction "denial." Unexpected things just seem to happen to addicts — they are buffeted by events rather than being in charge of their own lives. Their "early warning system" seems to be permanently turned off.

Co-addicts, too, do not trust themselves. They are so heavily invested in their relationship with the addict that, when given a choice between believing their own instincts and conclusions, versus something entirely different that the addict tells them, they all too often choose the addict's version over their own. Like addicts, co-addicts are in denial about what is happening around them. This is why they are often "the last to know" about their partner's affairs or other compulsive sexual behavior, even if the activities have been evident to the children, neighbors, and friends. Co-addicts are often completely unprepared when they learn about some hidden activity, even though there may have been many clues available. Not surprisingly, co-addicts find it difficult to trust others; their early warning system is also permanently inoperative, and if they cannot trust themselves, how could they possibly trust others?

People grow in their recovery from addiction and co-addiction when they learn to pay attention to the signals coming in from the outside world and to their own gut reactions. When individuals are able to trust themselves to use their own reactions as a guide to their responses, the world no longer seems so unpredictable. Events no longer "just happen." Instead, one feels a greater control of oneself. Learning to trust oneself is a prerequisite for negotiating the world with confidence and trust.

LAST WORDS

With its ability to transcend distance and facilitate social encounters between people, the Internet has revolutionized the social scene. The majority of Internet sex and relationship explorers have found this to be an enjoyable pastime that has enhanced their lives and brought new opportunities for dating and sexual exploration. However, a small percentage of online consumers are negatively affected. Ten years ago, cybersex addiction did not exist. Today, an ever-increasing number of people are getting hooked on Internet sex and experiencing significant negative consequences. Job performance drops in the workplace and people get fired. Marriages, committed relationships, health, family, self-care, and child care all are also affected.

This book discusses the consequences and describes the steps that those caught up in the Net can take to rebuild healthy lives. It explains the differences between recreational users of cybersex and its more problematic participants, allowing readers to position themselves and family members along the spectrum from recreation to addiction. By describing the steps to recovery from cybersex addiction and providing resources for those ready to get help, the authors wish to offer information and, most of all, hope to those who have lost parts of their lives and spirits to this addiction of isolation and loneliness. As with other addictions, those caught in the grip of cybersex addiction may feel hopeless and helpless. If you are among them, then you have taken the first step to hope and help by reading this book. Thousands recover daily from addictive behaviors by following the steps outlined here—recognizing their problem, going to a knowledgeable counselor, becoming involved in self-help groups, setting appropriate boundaries, rebuilding their relationships, and restoring balance to their lives. There *is* life after addiction. Addiction to cybersex can be conquered.

Three very different people describe, in their own words, the benefits of recovery from cybersex addiction:

Joe's Story: An At-Risk Cybersex User Pulls Back from the Brink

Joe was an outgoing thirty-four-year-old telephone salesman who'd been married for three years. In the past, he occasionally called a "900" telephone number and engaged in phone sex, more frequently in times of unusual stress. But he did not have a pattern of any compulsive sexual behaviors. When his job necessitated a move to a distant state, away from his family and friends, he went online and soon discovered sex chat rooms. Joe found himself spending more and more time chatting, which sometimes progressed to phone sex. He also got into exhibitionism and voyeurism using a digital video camera, both real-time with willing partners and through e-mail.

Meanwhile, Joe's relationship with his wife deteriorated. Their sex life became increasingly unsatisfying to him because he felt his online sex life was more imaginative and creative. It was equally unsatisfying for his wife, Ruth, because she sensed that he was more interested in sexual drama and variety than in simply being together and making love. They became emotionally distant and talked of separation. Joe made plans to meet an online romantic partner.

At the last moment, Joe and Ruth decided to stay together

and rebuild their relationship. Joe canceled his plans for a face-to-face meeting with the online partner. He ceased all cybersex activities. Even without formal counseling, the couple turned things around. Joe wrote:

> It's odd. The moment I diagnosed myself as an online sex addict, it stopped being difficult to abstain. I remember feeling as though an invisible opponent had suddenly become visible, and I could get in a couple of good punches where previously, I couldn't even see where to aim.
>
> I came up with some safety mechanisms but only had to use them a few times. Just getting out of the house and going to a movie helped. It did "waste" a few hours of my day, but that seemed better than potentially spending an entire day online. I still spend far too much time online, but none of that time is devoted to sexual activity.
>
> Sex with my wife has gotten better. It's still not as exciting as the thrill of exploring taboos, but it's more satisfying in the sense of not always craving something. I hope it continues to improve and that I'm able to increase my emotional connection.

Brenda's Story: Lifelong Consequences for a Female Sex Addict Hooked on the Net

Brenda, an attorney, grew up in a rigid and detached family, where mistakes were not tolerated and love was rarely given. The only affection she received was part of sexual abuse by a family member. Beginning in college and continuing for fifteen years thereafter, Brenda abused alcohol and engaged in anonymous sex, phone sex, pornography, and compulsive masturbation. She shares her story:

> When I finally landed in AA and had some knowledge of the Twelve Steps, I realized I was indeed powerless over my sex addiction. But it took three years on the Internet for me to hit

bottom and get help. I lost time, jobs, friends, money, and whatever self-respect I may have had.

I would go to work, race through my appointments, and as soon as possible, I would leave and go home. I'd get online, act out, go back to work, and again go home and get online as soon as I could. This went on for years. I was shut down emotionally. I'd get in a chat room looking for a man with whom I could have sex. I'd meet him at a hotel or at my house and have sex. When I traveled, I'd set up meetings in towns where I knew I would be staying. None of these meetings were ever romantic interests. I was clear from the beginning that it was about sex and nothing else. I also had pornographic sites that I frequented during those times when I was online but not in the chat room. Those sites mainly functioned to add to my file footage, which was continually running in my brain.

What got me offline was a frightening experience I had with a man whose house I'd gone to. I barely got out alive. I went home and put the computer in the car and drove it to a friend's house. I still want to get online—sometimes. I still want to get on the phone—sometimes. But I am in therapy now. I have a therapy group of wonderful people who have similar struggles. I have a wonderful therapist. I have a Twelve Step support group.

At a time in my life when I should have a spouse, family, and children, I have none of that. I have much regret and remorse for my actions. I grieve over what might have been in my life. However, I take full responsibility for my actions and the consequences of my behavior. Although it can be dark sometimes, I am on an exciting journey to redefine my spiritual life. I have good friends. I have taken on additional responsibilities at work. I am making more money. In short, I am getting my life back and attempting to regain a sense of self, character, and integrity.

*Thomas's Story: A Longtime Pornography Addict
Turns to the Internet*

Thomas was thirteen when he discovered pornography and masturbation. These activities continued to be an important part of his life, even after he got married. Thirty years later, he found something even better—the Internet—and within weeks it took over his life.

I became so engrossed in viewing porn photo files, reading erotic stories, and exchanging e-mails that nothing else really mattered. I lost time from work. I missed deadlines. I forgot family activities or dreaded them because they took me away from the computer. I neglected my former hobbies.

What I found on the computer was never enough. My appetite was never satisfied. One link led to many more. My standards for what are personally acceptable began to blur or vanish. I found myself enjoying materials that only a short time earlier would have been offensive or repulsive.

My relationship with my wife suffered. My sexual relationship with her became almost nonexistent. The sex we had was all self-centered for me. I found myself more comfortable with masturbation than with intercourse. Pornography went with me everywhere, in the form of printed stories to keep the rush going. Only when the rush was there did I feel temporarily free of the pain and guilt. I risked everything—job, wife, children, reputation—in pursuit of this compulsion.

When I recognized it as a compulsion, I knew I had a serious problem. But I did not and could not stop. It took a crisis situation to force me to confront my addiction: My oldest son found pornographic files on the computer and told his mother. In retrospect, this saved my marriage and job and made me turn my life around.

Through reading books such as *Out of the Shadows*, I recognized that I am a sex addict. I sought help through counseling and through a self-help program. I deleted all the pornographic bookmarks and files on my computer and destroyed all the printed matter related to this addiction. I rearranged my office so the computer is more visible from the door. I do not go back to the office after hours or stay late. I spend some time each day reading recovery material to remind myself of the nature of the problem and what I must do to avoid the traps and triggers. I do not use the computer at home unless someone else is there. I do not surf for sites to view. I begin and end each day in prayer that I may avoid the temptation and offer thanks for each day that I remain "free."

My wife and I have grown closer than ever after confronting the issues and learning the background causes. We have been talking a lot about everything. We read and study the same materials. We are learning how to have a healthy sexual relationship. She continues to be my strongest supporter, for which I will be forever grateful.

APPENDIX ONE

Resources

◘ ◘ ◘

THE TWELVE STEPS, MODIFIED FOR RECOVERY FROM COMPULSIVE SEXUAL BEHAVIORS*

1. We admitted we were powerless over sexual compulsion—that our lives had become unmanageable.

2. Came to believe that a power greater than ourselves could restore us to sanity.

3. Made a decision to turn our will and our lives over to the care of God, *as we understood God.*

4. Made a searching and fearless moral inventory of ourselves.

5. Admitted to God, to ourselves, and to another human being the exact nature of our wrongs.

6. Were entirely ready to have God remove all these defects of character.

7. Humbly asked God to remove our shortcomings.

8. Made a list of all persons we had harmed and became willing to make amends to them all.

9. Made direct amends to such people wherever possible, except when to do so would injure them or others.

183

10. Continued to take personal inventory and when we were wrong promptly admitted it.

11. Sought through prayer and meditation to improve our conscious contact with God, *as we understood God*, praying only for knowledge of God's will for us and the power to carry that out.

12. Having had a spiritual awakening as the result of these steps, we tried to carry this message to sexually compulsive people, and to practice these principles in all our affairs.

---

* Adapted from the Twelve Steps of Alcoholics Anonymous. Reprinted with permission of AA World Services, Inc., New York, N.Y. The Twelve Suggested Steps of SCA are taken from *Sexual Compulsives Anonymous: A Program of Recovery,* published by the International Service Organization of Sexual Compulsives Anonymous. (See editor's note on copyright page.)

THE TWELVE STEPS OF
ALCOHOLICS ANONYMOUS*

1. We admitted we were powerless over alcohol—that our lives had become unmanageable.

2. Came to believe that a Power greater than ourselves could restore us to sanity.

3. Made a decision to turn our will and our lives over to the care of God *as we understood Him.*

4. Made a searching and fearless moral inventory of ourselves.

5. Admitted to God, to ourselves, and to another human being the exact nature of our wrongs.

6. Were entirely ready to have God remove all these defects of character.

7. Humbly asked Him to remove our shortcomings.

8. Made a list of all persons we had harmed, and became willing to make amends to them all.

9. Made direct amends to such people wherever possible, except when to do so would injure them or others.

10. Continued to take personal inventory and when we were wrong promptly admitted it.

11. Sought through prayer and meditation to improve our conscious contact with God *as we understood Him,* praying only for knowledge of His will for us and the power to carry that out.

12. Having had a spiritual awakening as the result of these steps, we
    tried to carry this message to alcoholics, and to practice these
    principles in all our affairs.

---

* The Twelve Steps of AA are taken from *Alcoholics Anonymous*, 3d
  ed., published by AA World Services, Inc., New York, N.Y., 59–60.
  Reprinted with permission of AA World Services, Inc. (See editor's
  note on copyright page.)

SUGGESTED READING

I. Understanding and Recovering from Sex Addiction

Augustine Fellowship Staff. *Sex and Love Addicts Anonymous.* Boston: Sex and Love Addicts Anonymous, 1986. The official book of the fellowship of SLAA.

Carnes, Patrick. *Don't Call It Love: Recovery from Sexual Addiction.* New York: Bantam, 1991. Results of research on more than one thousand sex addicts.

Carnes, Patrick. *Out of the Shadows: Understanding Sexual Addiction.* Minneapolis: CompCare Publications, 1983. The groundbreaking book that explains sex addiction in easily understood terms.

Carnes, Patrick. *Sexual Anorexia: Overcoming Sexual Self-Hatred.* Center City, Minn.: Hazelden, 1997. The flip side of excessive sexual activities is avoiding sex while obsessing about it.

Earle, Ralph, and Gregory Crow. *Lonely All the Time: Recognizing, Understanding, and Overcoming Sex Addiction, for Addicts and Codependents.* New York: Pocket Books, 1989. Another easy-to-understand explanation of sex addiction.

Earle, Ralph, and Marcus Earle. *Sex Addiction: Case Studies and Management.* New York: Brunner Mazel, 1995. Good guide for therapists working with sex addicts.

Hazelden. *Hope and Recovery: A Twelve Step Guide for Healing from Compulsive Sexual Behavior.* Center City, Minn.: Hazelden, 1987. This recovery guide for sex addicts is modeled after the Big Book of Alcoholics Anonymous. It explains the problem and provides personal stories.

Kasl, Charlotte Davis. *Women, Sex, and Addiction: A Search for Love and Power.* New York: Ticknor and Fields, 1989. This book explores women sex addicts and women who hook up with sex addicts.

Sexaholics Anonymous. *Sexaholics Anonymous.* Simi Valley, Calif.: Sexaholics Anonymous, 1989. The official book of the fellowship of SA.

II. For Couples and for Families of Sex Addicts

Beattie, Melody. *Codependent No More: How to Stop Controlling Others and Start Caring for Yourself.* Center City, Minn.: Hazelden, 1986.

Carnes, Patrick. *The Betrayal Bond: Breaking Free of Exploitive Relationships.* Deerfield Beach, Fla.: Health Communications, 1997. This book shows how childhood trauma influences adult relationships.

Larsen, Earnie. *Stage II Relationships: Love Beyond Addiction.* San Francisco: Harper and Row, 1987. This book shows the importance of rebuilding relationships after Stage I recovery.

Norwood, Robin. *Women Who Love Too Much: When You Keep Wishing and Hoping He'll Change.* Los Angeles: Jeremy Tarcher, 1985. The classic book about women who get involved with addicts and how they can heal.

Schaeffer, Brenda. *Is It Love or Is It Addiction?* Second ed. Center City, Minn.: Hazelden, 1997. Useful for understanding healthy versus unhealthy relationships.

Schneider, Jennifer. *Back from Betrayal: Recovering from His Affairs.* Second ed. Tuscon, Ariz.: Recovery Resources Press, 2001. The classic book for women involved with sex-addicted men.

Schneider, Jennifer, and Burt Schneider. *Sex, Lies, and Forgiveness: Couples Speak on Healing From Sex Addiction.* Second ed. Tucson, Ariz.: Recovery Resources Press, 1999. A guide for couples who seek to rebuild their relationship.

Spring, Janis Abrahms. *After the Affair: Healing the Pain and Rebuilding Trust When a Partner Has Been Unfaithful.* New York: HarperCollins,

1996. No matter what the cause of the affair, this book describes how each party feels and how to recover.

Weiss, Douglas. *Partner's Recovery Guide: 100 Empowering Exercises.* Fort Worth, Tex.: Discovery Press, 1998. Helpful exercises for partners of sex addicts.

Weiss, Douglas, and Diane DeBusk. *Women Who Love Sex Addicts: Help for Healing from the Effects of a Relationship with a Sex Addict.* Fort Worth, Tex.: Discovery Press, 1993. A book for partners of sex addicts.

III. Internet Addiction and Cybersex Addiction

Fink, Jeri. *Cyberseduction: Reality in the Age of Psychotechnology.* Amherst, N.Y.: Prometheus Books, 1999. Gives an interesting explanation of why people are so attracted to virtual reality.

Greenfield, David D. *Virtual Addiction: Help for Netheads, Cyberfreaks, and Those Who Love Them.* Oakland, Calif.: New Harbinger Productions, 1999. Written in simple language, a book on how to break addictive connections to the Internet. There is some discussion of cybersex addiction.

Tarbox, Katherine. *Katie.com: My Story.* New York: Dutton, 2000. A first-person account of a young teen who inadvertently became involved online with a pedophile.

Young, Kimberly S. *Caught in the Net: How to Recognize the Signs of Internet Addiction—and a Winning Strategy for Recovery.* New York: John Wiley and Sons, 1998. This book explores the consequences of excessive involvement with Internet activities, but not cybersex.

IV. Sexuality

Barbach, Lonnie Garfield. *For Each Other: Sharing Sexual Intimacy.* Garden City, N.J.: Anchor Press, 1982.

Gochros, Jean, ed. *When Husbands Come Out of the Closet.* New York: Harrington Park Press, 1989.

Hunter, Mic. *Joyous Sexuality.* Minneapolis: CompCare Publications, 1992.

Maltz, Wendy. *The Sexual Healing Journey: A Guide for Survivors of Sexual Abuse.* San Francisco: HarperCollins, 1991.

THE MALE SEXUAL ADDICTION SCREENING TEST (G-SAST)

The Male Sexual Addiction Screening Test (G-SAST) is designed as a preliminary assessment screening for sexual addiction. The G-SAST provides a profile of responses that frequently help to identify men with sexual impulse disorders. To complete the test, answer each question by circling the appropriate answer. A score of eight or more suggests issues of sexual addiction, which would require further exploration with a professional clinician.

Yes No 1. Were you sexually abused as a child or adolescent?

Yes No 2. Have you subscribed to or regularly purchased/rented sexually explicit magazines or videos?

Yes No 3. Did your parents have trouble with their sexual or romantic behaviors?

Yes No 4. Do you often find yourself preoccupied with sexual thoughts?

Yes No 5. Has your use of phone sex lines, computer sex lines, etc., exceeded your ability to pay for these services?

Yes No 6. Does your significant other(s), friends, or family ever worry or complain about your sexual behavior? (Not related to sexual orientation.)

Yes No 7. Do you have trouble stopping your sexual behavior when you know it is inappropriate and/or dangerous to your health?

Yes No 8. Has your involvement with pornography, phone sex, computer board sex, etc., become greater than your intimate contacts with romantic partners?

Yes No   9. Do you keep the extent or nature of your sexual activities hidden from your friends and/or partners? (Not related to sexual orientation.)

Yes No   10. Do you look forward to events with friends or family being over so that you can go out to have sex?

Yes No   11. Do you visit sexual bathhouses, strip clubs, and/or video bookstores as a regular part of your sexual activity?

Yes No. 12. Do you believe that anonymous or casual sex has kept you from having more long-term intimate relationships or from reaching other personal goals?

Yes No   13. Do you have trouble maintaining intimate relationships once the "sexual newness" of the person has worn off?

Yes No   14. Do your sexual encounters place you in danger of arrest for lewd conduct or public indecency?

Yes No   15. Are you HIV positive, yet continue to engage in risky or unsafe sexual behavior?

Yes No   16. Has anyone ever been hurt emotionally by events related to your sexual behavior, for example, lying to partner or friends, not showing up for event/appointment due to sexual liaisons? (Not related to sexual orientation.)

Yes No   17. Have you ever been approached, charged, arrested by the police, security, etc., due to your sexual activities?

Yes No   18. Have you ever been sexual with a minor?

Yes No   19. When you have sex, do you feel depressed afterward?

Yes No   20. Have you made repeated promises to yourself to change some form of your sexual activity only to break them later? (Not related to sexual orientation.)

Yes No 21. Have your sexual activities interfered with some aspect of your professional or personal life, for example, unable to perform at work, loss of relationship? (Not related to sexual orientation.)

Yes No 22. Have you engaged in unsafe or "risky" sexual practices even though you knew it could cause you harm?

Yes No 23. Have you ever paid for sex?

Yes No 24. Have you ever had sex with someone just because you were feeling aroused and later felt ashamed or regretted it?

Yes No 25. Have you ever cruised public restrooms, rest areas, and/or parks looking for sexual encounters with strangers?

Developed by Robert Weiss, M.S.W., C.A.S., and Patrick J. Carnes, Ph.D., C.A.S.

WOMEN'S SEXUAL ADDICTION SCREENING TEST (W-SAST)

The Women's Sexual Addiction Screening Test (W-SAST) is designed to assist the assessment of sexually compulsive behavior. Depending on the particular pattern of symptoms, three positive answers may indicate an area of concern and should be discussed openly with a friend or family member. More than three positive answers would indicate the need to consider attending a Twelve Step support program such as Sex and Love Addicts Anonymous. Six or more true answers indicate an addictive problem with potentially self-abusive and/or dangerous consequences and indicate the need to seriously consider professional treatment.

1. Were you sexually abused as a child or adolescent?

2. Do you regularly purchase romance novels or sexually explicit magazines?

3. Have you stayed in romantic relationships after they have become emotionally or physically abusive?

4. Do you often find yourself preoccupied with sexual thoughts or romantic day dreams?

5. Do you feel that your sexual behavior is normal?

6. Does your spouse or significant other(s) ever worry or complain about your sexual behavior?

7. Do you have trouble stopping your sexual behavior when you know it is inappropriate?

8. Do you ever feel bad about your sexual behavior?

9. Has your sexual behavior ever created problems for you and your family?

10. Have you ever sought help for sexual behavior you did not like?

11. Have you ever worried about people finding out about your sexual activities?

12. Has anyone been hurt emotionally because of your sexual behavior?

13. Have you ever participated in sexual activity in exchange for money or gifts?

14. Do you have times when you act out sexually followed by periods of celibacy (no sex at all)?

15. Have you made efforts to quit a type of sexual activity and failed?

16. Do you hide some of your sexual behavior from others?

17. Do you find yourself having multiple romantic relationships at the same time?

18. Have you ever felt degraded by your sexual behavior?

19. Has sex or romantic fantasies been a way for you to escape your problems?

20. When you have sex, do you feel depressed afterwards?

21. Do you regularly engage in sado-masochistic behavior?

22. Has your sexual activity interfered with your family life?

23. Have you been sexual with minors?

24. Do you feel controlled by your sexual desire or fantasies of romance?

25. Do you ever think your sexual desire is stronger than you are?

By Patrick Carnes, Ph.D., and Sharon O'Hara, M.A.
(reprinted with permission)

CYBERSEX ADDICTION CHECKLIST

If you answer yes to three or more questions, this may be an area of concern and should be openly discussed with a friend or family member. If you answer yes to more than six questions, consider (a) counseling with a professional trained in addictive disorders and (b) checking out a Twelve Step support group for sexual addicts.

1. Are you spending increasing amounts of online time on sexual or romantic intrigue or involvement?

2. Have you been involved in multiple online romantic or sexual affairs?

3. Do you prefer online sex to having "real" sex with your spouse or primary partner?

4. Have you tried unsuccessfully to cut back on the time you spend online in sexual and romantic activities?

5. Has the time you spend in online sex or romance interfered with your job or other important commitments?

6. Have you collected a large quantity of Internet pornography?

7. Have you engaged in fantasy online acts or experiences which would be illegal if carried out (e.g., rape or sex with children or adolescents)?

8. Has your online sexual or romantic involvement resulted in spending significantly less time with your spouse/partner, dating life, or friends?

9. Have you lied about the amount of time you spend online or the type of sexual or romantic activities you experience online?

10. Have you had sexual experiences online that you wish to keep hidden from a partner or spouse?

11. Have your family or friends increasingly complained or been concerned about the amount of time you have spent online?

12. Do you frequently become angry or very irritable when asked to get off the Internet or off the computer?

13. Has the computer become the primary focus of your sexual or romantic life?

Robert Weiss, M.S.W., C.A.S.

NATIONAL TWELVE STEP SEXUAL
RECOVERY MEETING INFORMATION

The following list briefly describes sexual recovery programs, their focus, and their attendance. Contact the national offices by phone or visit their Web sites for more specific meeting information, locations, and times.

Addict and Offender Groups

SA—Sexaholics Anonymous. A national Twelve Step program, employing a conservative definition of *sexual sobriety:* "No sexual behavior outside of a marital relationship." The membership of this group is primarily heterosexual men, but an increasing number of women attend. SA has an affiliated program for spouses and families of sex addicts and offenders called S-Anon. Heterosexual men who are in a committed, married relationship would benefit most from the recovery materials available from this fellowship. This organization tends to attract and serve a more conservative addict population because of the predefined nature of its sobriety definition. The sex offender population is also more heavily represented in SA for this same reason. Some people consider SA to be less supportive of sexual orientations other than heterosexual. Newcomers and old-timers alike, as well as people who speak Spanish or German, can find resources. SA is also the only Twelve Step group that offers a program for prisoners. Spouses will find links for family members on SA's Web site.
Web site: **www.sa.org**
E-mail address: saico@sa.org
Phone: (615) 331-6230
Fax: (615) 331-6901

SAA—Sex Addicts Anonymous. A national Twelve Step program that encourages participants to define their sexual sobriety through working with other recovering members. Attendance is mixed, primarily men of both sexual orientations with some limited female attendance. SAA has an affiliated program for partners of sexual addicts called COSA (Codependents of Sex Addicts).

Web site: **www.sexaa.org**

E-mail address: info@saa-recovery.org

Phone: (713) 869-4902

SCA—Sexual Compulsives Anonymous. A Twelve Step program found in major urban areas. Membership is heavily gay and bisexual men and some women. Participants define their sexual sobriety through the boundaries of a written plan that evolves through working with other recovering members. SCA has no formal partners program. People with differing sexual orientations would find this program most beneficial.

Web site: **www.sca-recovery.org**

E-mail address: info@sca-recovery.org

Telephone: (800) 977-4325

SLAA—Sex and Love Addicts Anonymous. This Twelve Step program focuses on addictive sexual and romantic relationships. SLAA is helpful for sexual addicts as well as people who consistently involve themselves in abusive, non-nurturing relationships. This program attracts both men and women. SLAA is the most broadly supportive of women of all the Twelve Step sexual addictions organizations. What differentiates this group is that it focuses on the recovery from problems related to romantic dependency, romantic relationships, emotional dependency, and social or emotional anorexia.

Web site: **www.slaahouston.org**

E-mail address: slaafws@aol.com

Phone: (781) 255-8825

SRA—Sexual Recovery Anonymous. This is a "non-Higher Power" Twelve Step program for sex addicts and sex offenders modeled after Rational Recovery, which focuses on spirituality and self-love rather than the notion of a "Higher Power." SRA meetings are limited in number but open to all in sexual recovery. This organization is somewhat limited in scope, with scattered meetings in the New

York–Connecticut–New Jersey tri-state area as well as Los Angeles, Atlanta, and Vancouver, Canada.
Web site: **www.ourworld.compuserve.com/homepages/sra**
Phone: (212) 340-4650

Partner and Couple Groups

S-Anon. A national Twelve Step program for partners and families of sex addicts and sex offenders. Although primarily married women attend, there are also many single members. The fellowship welcomes anyone whose life has been affected in the present or past by a relationship with a sex addict. S-Anon is affiliated with SA and supports S-Ateen, a program for children of sex addicts.
Web site: **www.sanon.org**
E-mail: Sanon@sanon.org
Phone: (615) 833-3152

COSA—Codependents of Sex Addicts. A national Twelve Step program for partners and significant others of sex addicts and sex offenders. The fellowship is affiliated with SAA. Anyone who is in a relationship with a sexual addict is welcome. Because of the links available to the family groups, this Web site makes it easy for spouses and other family members to find appropriate groups for their recovery. One option made available through this organization is online meetings. Information describing what an online meeting is, how to join one, a listing of current online meetings, and how to start an online meeting is clearly laid out.
Web site: **www.shore.net/~cosa**
E-mail: cosa@shore.net
Phone: (612) 537-6904

RCA—Recovering Couples Anonymous. A newer Twelve Step program that helps both addicts and their partners work on issues of commitment, intimacy, and mutual recovery. All couples—married, non-married, gay, and straight—are welcome. The fellowship is open to couples dealing with any addiction.

Web site: **www.recovering-couples.org**
E-mail: RCAWSO@1name.com
Phone: (314) 397-0867

ABOUT ONLINE/WEB SITE RESOURCES

Each Web site listed above offers information primarily as outreach to new and current members, providing information, support services, and links to related organizations. The Web sites can be viewed from all current browsers. They all appear easy to understand and are user friendly. Several of the sites have online meetings, a feature of particular value to those either geographically or physically unable to attend actual support meetings. These online meetings are hosted and managed by the particular support group; therefore the content of the discussions is maintained within appropriate boundaries. Participation in the online meetings requires the use of software specific to that site. Each online meeting host site provides the links needed to obtain the required software.

OTHER SUPPORTIVE RESOURCES

The National Council on Sexual Addiction and Compulsivity (NCSAC). This is a private, nonprofit organization dedicated to the promotion of public and professional recognition, awareness, and understanding of sexual addiction, sexual compulsivity, and sexual offending. NCSAC is an educational and referral resource for sex addicts, sexual offenders, and any counseling, criminal justice, or research professional in need of information or referrals, and for the media. The Web site of NCSAC, **www.ncsac.org**, contains position papers, national referrals, and information about the annual national conference.

www.SexHelp.com. Dr. Patrick Carnes's Resources for Sex Addiction and Recovery, offers addiction and recovery resources from international sex addiction expert Patrick Carnes, Ph.D. It features the leading books, videos, and audios in the field of sex addiction and recovery.

The Healthy Mind. This Web site, **www.healthymind.com**, by clinical psychologist David Bissette, from Washington, D.C., offers information about sex addiction and how to recover from it. Pages include both explanations about the nature of addiction and worksheets for establishing and maintaining sobriety.

Sexual Addiction Recovery Resources. Useful for addicts, co-addicts (spouses, significant others, and friends), and counselors, **www. home.rmi.net/~slg/sarr** contains links to various sex addiction recovery-related resources on the Internet.

Online Sexual Addiction: Education, Support, and Resources. This Web site, **www.onlinesexaddict.com**, is dedicated to providing education, support, and resources to people concerned about their own or others' compulsive sexual behavior on the World Wide Web.

The Center for On-Line Addiction. A training institute and behavioral heath care firm specializing in Internet-related conditions such as problem day trading, compulsive online shopping, gambling, online infidelity, cybersexual addiction, and the social dangers of computers to children. Established by Dr. Kimberly Young, this institute's professional services include outpatient therapy, forensic evaluations, health care, and corporate training. The center also offers a virtual clinic that provides e-mail, chat rooms, and telephone counseling. For more information contact Dr. Young at ksy@netaddiction.com or call (814) 362-7045.

The Sexual Recovery Institute (SRI). A therapy agency specializing in the elimination of compulsive sexual behaviors. Persons with issues such as multiple affairs, compulsive use of pornography, phone and cybersex, anonymous sex, compulsive masturbation, sexual massage/prostitution, exhibitionism/voyeurism, and perpetrators of sexual harassment make up the client base. Established by Robert Weiss, M.S.W., C.A.S., the agency provides outpatient assessment and treatment to southern Californians and offers extended intensive treatment to visitors from other areas. The institute also provides professional training and national referral. For more information, contact SRI at **www.sexualrecovery.com** or call (310) 360-0130.

APPENDIX TWO

Avoiding the Pitfalls of Internet Dating

◼ ◻ ◼

Both e-mail and chat rooms use the written language for communication. While such correspondence has many advantages, as discussed earlier, one downside is that it eliminates important information relevant to choosing a romantic partner. Gender, age, profession, and any other characteristics can be misrepresented. The person online may turn out to be very different in the real world. Online romances can be idealized fantasies with very little connection to reality. Yet for many people the Internet is a very positive tool for gathering information, communicating with friends, and establishing healthy romantic relationships. These people's experiences can serve as positive role models for healthy dating on the Internet. Consider the story of Joan, who found herself single in middle age.

> Two years after her twenty-year marriage ended, Joan was finally ready to begin dating. As a fifty-year-old physician, she was not very optimistic about her chances of meeting a compatible man: She lived in a fairly small community, did not like the bar scene, and ethics precluded her from dating the only people she encountered at work, her patients. There were a few traditional matchmakers in the community, but their fees were exorbitant and their success rate small. A friend suggested that she enroll in an online matchmaking service. To her surprise, within a month she had blind dates with several very nice, sincere, professional men. She and her dates all led isolated lives that provided scant opportunities for meeting

dating partners—and the Internet had suddenly greatly expanded their options. Within weeks Joan found Jay, a compatible man whose company she enjoyed.

Like Joan, Stan, a fifty-year-old architect, also found himself alone:

Stan's wife of many years had developed a progressive disease that increasingly put him in a caretaker role. He found help and understanding in an e-mail support group for families of people with the same disease. After his wife's death, Stan continued corresponding with several members of the same online support group, including Rose, whose husband had also just died. Stan and Rose eventually met in person, and a year later they got engaged.

Unfortunately, as discussed earlier, Internet interaction does have its downside. The absence of the sensory cues—sight, sound, touch, smell—provides greater opportunities for deception. Surveys show that a large proportion of people lie about themselves on the Internet. Most commonly, they favorably alter their age, height, or weight, or post a picture of themselves that was taken five or more years earlier. Some people claim to be of the opposite gender—gender bending—they pretend to be teenagers when they are in fact middle-aged adults, or they disguise their predatory intent. If one becomes interested in meeting a dating partner through the Internet, it makes sense to be self-protective. Following are some things to consider.

INTENTIONS

Susie longed to meet "Mr. Right," a caring man who would sweep her off her feet and marry her. She met Brandon in a sexually oriented chat room. Initially they exchanged sexual messages and subsequently had sex online using video-streaming. Finally they met offline and began an intense sexual relationship. Susie thought she had met her dream man. After a year of seeing each other, she was devastated to learn that Brandon was continuing to have sex with several other women on the computer.

Susie should not have been surprised. People who frequent erotic or sexual chat rooms generally do so for the purpose of finding sexual partners, not life partners. If you are looking for a dating partner with similar interests, you are more likely to meet him or her on a legitimate dating site or a general-interest chat room (bicycles, travel, music, or books).

Although most people who sign up on dating sites are legitimate, a few are not. When visiting dating sites, read their anonymity statement and use caution. Below are some online dating services that are not specifically sexually oriented. We do not specifically recommend or endorse any of them.

- **Match.com**
- **Matchmaker.com**
- **Jdate.com** (Jewish singles)
- **PlanetOut.com** (Gay and Lesbian)
- **Rightstuffdating.com** (graduates of selected universities)
- AOL, Compuserve, Earthlink, MSN, and other ISPs' "Personals" and "Dating" areas

SAFETY

Although the individuals at the other end of the keyboard may seem friendly and well-intentioned, it is impossible to know initially whether they really are who they represent themselves to be. It is prudent, therefore, not to disclose addresses, telephone numbers, financial status, or work circumstances. The safest dating sites are those that forward e-mail using a different e-mail address. When using a screen name to enroll in a dedicated dating site, the person being contacted doesn't know a real name or actual e-mail address. There are also dating sites that do not list e-mail addresses within profiles, but if someone wants to be in contact, the dating service supplies the actual e-mail address. A dating service that includes one's own e-mail address on screen is the least safe. When providing a self-description in online profiles, focus on interests and personality characteristics. Do not reveal your address, your place of employment, a six-figure income, and other personal life details.

After several e-mail exchanges, you may feel comfortable enough to give out your telephone number and have a phone conversation. It's a good idea to get the other person's telephone number as well, and call him or her. People who are married or lying about other important matters are less likely to give out their phone number.

If choosing to meet in person, public places are best. Telling another friend of your specific arrangement is a good idea. If traveling a long distance to meet someone, it is ideal to have return arrangements in place, meet in a public place, and again advise a friend or family member of the exact plans and schedule.

If meeting someone in a general interest chat room or a dating site (as opposed to a sexually oriented location), there is reason to be concerned if the person asks intrusive or peculiar questions, seeks sexual information, or wants a phone number without disclosing his or hers. For example, in the book *Katie.com*, the story of a thirteen-year-old girl who inadvertently became involved with "Vallleyguy," a forty-two-year-old pedophile, his very first question to her in an online teenage chat room was, "How old is the oldest person you will speak to online?" "Twenty-seven," she replied. He then wrote, "That's good, because I'm only twenty-three. What is your age/sex?" She wrote, "Thirteen/F." At the end of the exchange, he asked for her phone number, without giving his. Soon thereafter, he asked her if she was a virgin and expressed an interest in flying to her city to meet her. When they finally met in a hotel room out of town, she narrowly escaped being sexually assaulted.

Rather than communicating directly with children online, other pedophiles target women who have children of the desired age. If a man seems more interested in your children than you, consider it a red flag.

Also be forewarned about people who are reluctant to divulge details of their life while probing you for yours, or who give you conflicting information about crucial aspects of their life, such as marital status, career, family circumstances, or financial status.

Sooner or later, people who are getting to know each other online exchange photos. In helping a subscriber decide whether or not to post a photograph with her online profile, **match.com** reports that those who post a photo online get three times as many inquiries as those who don't. Obviously, posting your photograph makes you less anonymous, so some people choose to wait until they are exchanging e-mails with someone.

THE MASK OF ONLINE COMMUNICATION

Communicating by e-mail is like exchanging regular letters (known by computer folk as "snail mail"), only they are transmitted much faster via the Internet than by trucks, airplanes, or the friendly mail carrier. E-mail can be accessed at one's convenience, allowing all the time needed to compose a well-thought-out and well-written reply. Unfortunately, e-mail provides few clues about the person since visual and auditory cues are absent.

One alternative to e-mail is the chat room, which allows for real-time conversation among a group of people, using the medium of typing rather than speech. A variant of the chat room is the private room, where people can converse by typing instant messages to each other. Written exchanges occur much faster in chat rooms or private rooms than they do with e-mail, so there may be more revealed about the person's personality. Of course, telephone conversations give even more information—allowing a vocal impression as well as clues about the other person's ability to listen and empathize. Nothing, however, beats a face-to-face meeting. Many have had the experience of meeting someone for the first time and of knowing within a few minutes that the person was someone they do—or don't—want to see again. Often this is a response to the many visual, emotional, and intuitive cues people unconsciously receive. Despite having exchanged a hundred e-mails or having spent many enjoyable hours on the phone with someone, there may be a strong negative reaction on an initial face-to-face meeting. All those hours on the computer (and the phone) suddenly seem like a disappointing waste of time.

The relative anonymity of the computer can foster a pseudo-intimacy, encouraging people to reveal themselves in ways they might not in a real-life meeting. This perceived sense of trust and acceptance leads to the illusion that they know each other very well, whereas in fact they may hardly know each other at all. In some cases, the longer the couple has been relating long-distance on this intimate level, the more daunting is the possibility of a face-to-face meeting. The result may be that a person passes up a real-life relationship by spending hours alone on the computer, pursuing a long-term online pseudo-intimate relationship with someone they've never met. In order to prevent disappointment, some people avoid an actual meeting. Rather than risk the demise of the relationship, a face-to-face meeting may be postponed indefinitely.

To avoid these obstacles, it is important to define the goal of meeting someone online. If, for example, it is to acquire a support system to help work through a life crisis or that of a family member (such as an illness), then online friendships may be the perfect answer. But if the goal is a dating relationship with the possibility of intimacy, then the Internet becomes most useful as an initial screening tool. If your goal is a romantic relationship, avoid a long-term online-only friendship. Once it is established that this is someone safe and interesting enough to get to know better, arrange an offline meeting.

APPENDIX THREE

Frequently Asked Questions about Sex Addiction and Cybersex Addiction

■ ▣ ▣

Q: I spend many hours a week online in cybersex activities and I enjoy every moment. How do I know if I am a sex addict?

The primary way to identify any addictive behavior is to consider whether it is causing negative or unwelcome problems in your life and yet you return to it anyway. If your sexual behaviors have caused consequences to your legal status, relationships, career, health (emotional or physical), yet you continue to engage in those sexual behaviors, then there is likely a problem. You know that you are a cybersex addict if your computer-based sexual behaviors take up more time, energy, and focus than you would like or if they cause you to act in ways that go against your underlying values and beliefs.

Men and women who are addicts frequently say to themselves, "This is the last time that I am going to . . ." yet they find themselves driven to return to the same sexual situations despite previous commitments to change. Cybersex addicts are often unable to make and keep commitments to themselves and others about stopping or changing particular sexual behaviors over the long term, and most have problems with real intimacy. They describe having feelings of overwhelming intensity while approaching a situation in which they may participate in their particular sexual behavior, and describe this intensity state as "being in the bubble" or "like being in a trance."

This intensity/arousal state is typical and allows sex addicts to block out the potential consequences of what they are about to do. Typical sexual addict behaviors include compulsive use of the Internet, phone lines, or personals ads for sex; consistent use of prostitutes, sexual massage, or escorts; multiple affairs; frequent sex outside of primary relationships; anonymous sex; and compulsive masturbation.

Q: If I turn out to be a cybersex addict, why can't I just take prescription medications to reduce my sex drive?

Certain antidepressant drugs (such as Prozac, Paxil, and Celexa) can reduce sexual drive and also can be extremely helpful for the anxiety and depressive symptoms that can underlie many addictive behaviors, but these medications alone do not solve the problems underlying sex addiction. Male hormone-suppressing medications are used primarily in the treatment of sex offenders to help dampen their obsessive preoccupation with illegal sexual activity. However, these drugs are effective only as long as they are being used and do not produce permanent changes to compulsive sexual behaviors.

For cybersex addicts, long-term addiction-based counseling, Twelve Step support group attendance, and a commitment to making adjustments in life circumstances are the best start toward creating long-term change. Sexual addiction is not about just being too horny or wanting sex too often. It is a disorder in which cruising, flirting, fantasy, intrigue, and sex itself are used as ways of managing and tolerating feelings and underlying emotional conflicts. Cybersex addicts seek sexual highs to substitute for the support and intimacy they really need but do not allow themselves to have. Even though they may be surrounded by friends, family, or supportive spouses, sex addicts will turn to the isolating intensity of their sexual behaviors for comfort rather than using the available real human support. Recovering from any type of sex addiction is more than a physical problem that can be solved by taking a pill; it also involves complex and often confusing emotional concerns.

Q: The sexual behaviors that I most often engage in are masturbation with pornography. Can this be a part of sex addiction?

Yes. Compulsive masturbation with or without pornography and compulsive viewing of porn with or without masturbation both present long-standing problems for many cybersex addicts. Whether it is through cybersex, phone sex lines, videos, porn magazines, or simply through fantasy, sex addicts can lose hours daily to the isolating activities of fantasy and masturbation.

Cybersex addiction in particular does not necessarily involve having skin-to-skin contact with another partner, thereby making it safer for those sex addicts too afraid of getting caught, catching a disease, or being rejected to seek out partners for their acting out. Those involved in compulsive masturbation or compulsive viewing of online or other pornography may lead lonely, disconnected lives, never really understanding what keeps them from real intimacy and connection with other people. Other sex addicts may be married or in a primary relationship, yet prefer masturbation to having sex with their available and willing partner.

Many cybersex addicts who use compulsive masturbation as their primary way of sexual acting out are in complete denial that their patterns of sexual release are any different from most people. Caught in compulsive patterns—often begun in childhood or adolescence—the person who is masturbating compulsively may masturbate every night to get to sleep or every morning while showering. These behaviors become as much a part of their daily routine as eating or sleeping.

Q: If alcoholics and drug addicts define "being sober" by not drinking or using mind-altering chemicals, how does a cybersex addict define sobriety—abstaining from sex altogether?

Unlike sobriety from the use of mood-altering substances, sexual sobriety is not usually defined as abstinence from sex, although some recovering people may take a short period of abstinence or celibacy to help gain personal perspective or address a particular issue. Sexual sobriety is most often defined through the use of a "sexual recovery plan" or "contract" between the sex addict and his or her Twelve Step recovery support sponsor, therapist, or clergy. These plans are ideally written down and involve clearly defined, concrete behaviors from which the addict commits to abstain. Some relationship or sexual recovery plans have very strictly defined boundaries, such as no sexual activity of any kind outside of a committed marital relationship or no sex before being in a committed relationship.

Sobriety is defined as abstinence from the identified sexual and cybersexual activities that cause the addict to feel shameful or hold secrets, or that are illegal or abusive. Personal definitions may change over time as recovering individuals evolve in their understanding of the disease. One recovering man's early contract started out as, "I am sober as long as I do not have sex in public places, use Internet pornography or chat rooms, see prostitutes or old girlfriends (whom I am just seeing for the sexual contact)." This man's "sex plan" evolved over the period of a few months to be all of the above plus: "I am sober as long as I do not engage in flirtation, intrigue, or sexual seduction with strangers or have sexual or romantic liaisons with anyone I have dated for less than ninety days. I do not meet sexual or romantic partners over the Internet." Contracts such as these are created in concert with at least one other recovering person, therapist, or clergy, and are not altered without the prior agreement of those trusted people.

Q: My wife caught me several months ago in online cybersex/ romantic chats and porn viewing. At the time, I admitted I had a problem and joined a Twelve Step program for help. I have not acted out sexually since that time. However, she continues to be distant, critical, angry, and mistrustful. What can I do to make our relationship improve?

This situation is frequently encountered by newly recovering cybersex addicts. Despite the recovering addict's solid recovery program and no slips, the partner remains angry, devaluing, and distant.

Although you are doing well and dealing with the issues, and deserve lots of support and validation, it seems wrong to ask that your partner be the one to offer you that validation right now. As with many recovering sex addicts, you are missing the relationship side of the issue. How can your partner be sure that you are no longer betraying your relationship and that you have now decided to keep your part of the relationship bargain? Put in that context, it can be easier to understand that your partner is deeply hurt, angry, and suspicious. Your wife probably will remain that way for some time. Just as she stood by as you emotionally abandoned the relationship through your cybersexual acting out, you will have to be patient with her anger, disappointment, and suspicion. It is vital that she express those feelings, even if they are hurtful, difficult, and sometimes intolerable to you.

As a consequence of your previous actions, your couple relationship will experience challenges for quite a while. It can take up to two years for partners to overcome their hurt and sense of betrayal, to forgive, and to rebuild trust. In the meantime, you need the support for the difficult work of recovery that can be found with friends in Twelve Step programs, sponsors, and therapists. Give your partner space and understanding to express his or her hurt and anger without trying to avoid it, dismiss it, or make it different. In time, things will improve. It is always helpful to consider couples counseling, attending Recovering Couples Anonymous (RCA) or other couples' support groups to help work through the rough times. (See appendix 1 for a list of such programs.)

Q: For many years I have found ways to satisfy what I have always perceived as a large sexual appetite. My partner doesn't seem to want to have a lot of sex, so I have been involved in affairs, both online and offline, use porn, and regularly receive sensual massages. Is this really a problem?

One of the first questions to ask yourself in determining whether you have a sexual addiction or cybersex problem is, "Why am I even asking myself about the appropriateness of my sexual behavior?" Most people don't consistently question whether what they are doing sexually is right for them, nor do most people use the comments of "locker room conversations" to justify or compare their own sexual activities to others'. It is worth noting that even asking these kinds of questions may indicate that deep down you think there is some kind of problem.

Second, part of what determines whether someone is a sex addict is not just looking at the person's sexual behaviors, but also at how he or she is living his or her life. Many sex addicts constantly lie to their partners, keep sexual secrets, and find ways to justify their sexual behaviors. How does your current sex life affect your sense of integrity and your own personal values or belief systems? How does it make you look at yourself? Regardless of what others say they do, how do you feel about your sexual behavior, and is it a secret? It is one thing if you and your spouse agree that some of your sexual activity will take place outside of the relationship, but are you sneaking around using lies or omissions to get away with your activities?

As to the sex itself, a sex addict is someone who engages in persistent and escalating patterns of sexual behaviors despite harmful consequences or potential consequences to self or others. This means that for the sex and cybersex addict, the sexual behaviors in question either have caused serious consequences to life (legal, relationship, career, emotional, physical, and so on) or that they have the potential to do so, and yet those risks are being ignored.

Before deciding whether you are a sex addict, ask yourself if you are ignoring life consequences in order to maintain access to your sexual activities. One thing that can help determine if there is a sex addiction problem is to simply take a time-out from all sexual behavior. Attempt to not have sex at all for thirty days and see:

1. Can you keep the commitment?
2. How difficult was keeping it?
3. What feelings and experiences did you have while taking this time-out?

If you cannot maintain the commitment to yourself or find it extremely difficult, you may have a problem. Also, consider attending some sex addiction Twelve Step programs to get a clearer idea of the problem and how to manage it.

Q: I am a gay man who has had multiple sexual encounters in bathhouses and sex clubs, as well as meeting anonymous sex partners through online chats. I am having trouble with calling myself a sex addict. I have gone through a lifetime of feeling stigmatized for my sexual orientation. Now it seems that by considering myself a "sex

addict," I am just adding to that stigma. Although I do struggle with the nature and degree of my sexual behaviors, I wonder whether the label of sex addiction is just another way of making me wrong for my sexuality.

It is very understandable that you would not want to be the subject of a cultural prejudice any more than you have already been, but there are some important points that you should keep in mind. Being a sex addict is not something that *anyone* wants or chooses. There is no difference between a straight sex addict and a gay sex addict except the sex of the person whom they are pursuing. Straight men have strip bars, prostitutes, adult movie theaters, porn, and cybersex. Gay men have sex clubs, bathhouses, prostitutes, adult movies, porn, and cybersex. The choices are slightly different, but the behavior is exactly the same. If you sit and listen to both straight and gay sex addicts speak about their problems, you quickly find that they have more in common in terms of the intensity, drive, and compulsive nature of their behaviors than they have differences. The best sex addiction recovery work is done when sex addicts are able to reach below superficial differences to see those commonalities.

Acknowledging that you may be a sex addict does not attach a negative label to your morality, value system, or humanity, no more than would calling someone who drinks to excess an alcoholic. The "label" of sex addiction is simply the most convenient and accurate term to describe certain sets of compulsive sexual behaviors that need a particular kind of treatment. There is no clinical judgment placed on the diagnosis or the treatment of sex addiction, though feelings of shame, fear, and embarrassment about being a sex addict are perfectly normal and predictable.

Q: I am a married woman and my time online is mostly spent in sex and romance chats. I keep a secret screen name so I can carry on my computer sex activities without my husband finding out. I've had brief offline affairs with some of these men. I am afraid and embarrassed to ask for help. Most everything I read and see about sex addicts refers to men and their behaviors. This makes me feel like a

woman can't have this problem, or she has to be even sicker to have it. Yet, I think I am a sex addict and I really struggle with this.

There are many women sex addicts. The problem is not as common or obvious for women as for men, but that doesn't mean that there aren't many women who suffer from compulsive sexual and romantic behaviors. You hit on a major reason why so few women feel comfortable admitting a sex addiction problem. After all, what do we call a man who frequently acts out with sexual conquests and sexualized behavior? Stud, macho, dude, or just plain "lucky" are the kinds of names most often applied to men in this category. But what of women who frequently engage in sexual activity? Our culture calls them sluts, whores, loose—not exactly the kind of validation that anyone would want. So, while our society often rewards men for excessive sexual behavior, it simultaneously punishes and devalues women for the same activities. No wonder it is so difficult for women to come forth and admit they have a problem.

About sixty years ago or so when AA (Alcoholics Anonymous) was getting started, most of those meetings were male dominated. Alcoholics were assumed to be males, usually found drunk in back alleys and halfway houses. Of course, now we know there were many women alcoholics too. They were just more likely to be at home tipping the cooking sherry than out in a bar getting publicly drunk. The same situation applies to sexual recovery. Males today dominate most sexual recovery meetings, though this is beginning to change.

Increasingly, Twelve Step sexual recovery programs are opening themselves and their membership to women, some providing women-only sessions while others offer more mixed support meetings. It is essential that women in sexual recovery seek out and find the fellowship of other recovering women to share their stories and reduce the stigma of being a woman with this problem.

Q. My partner is spending more and more time late at night on the computer in his study, and less and less time with me. We used to have an active sex life, but it's been three months since we made

love even once. Last month he bought some new gadgets for the computer, including a digital camera. I suspect he's spending nights viewing pornography online and maybe even meeting people for sex. I asked him about this and he denied it. I'm sick at heart, but I just don't know what to do.

Whether or not your partner is indeed engaging in cybersex, your relationship is in trouble. Your sex life has disappeared, your time together has diminished, and your trust in him has eroded. It's clearly time for some damage control and some honest discussions about what is happening. Go together to see a couples counselor, preferably one who is knowledgeable about how the Internet can affect relationships. If your partner is unwilling to go, then it is very likely that he is hiding some behavior. In this case, it would be helpful for you to see a counselor alone in order to sort out your options. You might also consider joining an online support group for partners of sex addicts. The only requirement for membership is that you are being affected by someone else's sexual behavior. These days, cybersex addiction is a major topic of discussion on the online support groups.

Q. Ten months ago I caught my husband having real-time sex with a woman online. He later admitted to me that he'd been involved in cybersex for years. Now he says he's stopped and is in recovery from sex addiction. I know he's really trying—he's always at Twelve Step meetings, on the phone with other recovering people, and so on. I want to trust him again, but somehow I can't. I feel betrayed and angry. I also feel unattractive—I look nothing like those cybersex women. He says he never had a "real" affair and doesn't understand why I can't just let go of the past and forgive him. Whenever I look at the computer, I get upset all over again.

People who've had to deal with a spouse who's had real-time online sex report that it feels just as painful as an offline affair. They feel just as betrayed, cheated on, discounted, and lied to. Your husband may believe he didn't have a real affair, but you are not the only one who feels that he committed just another form of adultery. It might help for both of you to go to a knowledgeable counselor to discuss your feelings. Consider going to meetings of RCA (Recovering Couples Anonymous) to learn how other couples have coped. Or get together with another couple who've had a similar experience and ask them what has worked for them.

Cybersex is fantasy sex. A real sex partner, no matter how attractive, just can't measure up to the fantasy women online. It is natural for real-life partners of cybersex addicts to compare themselves unfavorably to the cyberwomen, to wonder if they could ever measure up, and to feel a loss of self-esteem. Counseling and a support group can help you realize that your husband's past preference for fantasy women is his problem and says nothing about your own attractiveness or lack of it.

Forgiveness can be defined as being able to remember the past without feeling pain all over again. An addict in recovery is often impatient and, like your husband, thinks that ten months is more than enough time to rebuild trust. In the aftermath of an affair, it typically takes two years for the betrayed partner to truly forgive and let go of what happened, even if the recovering addict is toeing the line and working a good recovery program.

Rebuilding trust occurs most rapidly when the addict is committed to recovery and demonstrates this by continued involvement in counseling and Twelve Step groups; when the addict is honest, regarding both little and big things, day after day; and when the partner is also involved in counseling and a self-help group.

Usually, when someone in a committed relationship has had an affair, it is easier for the spouse to begin to trust the unfaithful partner again if he or she agrees to end all contact with that sexual partner. If the person remains on the scene (for example, a next-door neighbor or a co-worker), it is much harder for the deceived partner to feel safe again. In the case of cybersex addiction, in which the home computer played a major role, the continuing presence of the computer in the home can delay the spouse's healing. Consider removing the computer from the home for at least a few weeks, until its presence no longer feels like reopening a wound. One day you'll be able to look at the computer, remember the bad days that it symbolizes, but not feel any pain.

Q. After the intensity and novelty of cybersex, can sex with an ordinary long-term partner ever be just as good?

Most people in long-term relationships remember the excitement of the first weeks and months when they were newlyweds or just beginning their sexual relationship. In most cases, as they get to know each other better and have hundreds of nights of lovemaking together, the intensity diminishes along with the novelty. Ideally, what develops out of that initial intensity is a deeper and more meaningful sense of intimacy and trust. The lure of affairs is that they offer the opportunity to once again experience that level of excitement and intensity in sex. Yet most people who are in committed long-term relationships spend very little time in sex outside of their primary relationship. The reasons are that the gifts offered within a committed relationship are so meaningful, and the sex can continue to be very good even after many years. The price to pay for an affair is considered to be too high by most people.

Cybersex gives the participant a concentrated dose of those early intensity-based days of sex in a new relationship. The availability of these intense experiences makes the Internet so seductive. But cybersex has many drawbacks as well, and the price can be exorbitant. Sex on the Internet feels incomplete to the many people who push for real-life meetings with their cybersex partners; there is no substitute for skin-to-skin contact. Alone with only the computer for company, cybersex participants are in fact isolated from real human contact. Cybersex objectifies the participants. They are often reduced to body parts. Real-life sex with a committed partner can create an intimacy that makes it much better than sex with one's own hand and a picture on a screen, yet this intimacy also involves a degree of self-sacrifice and risk. Real-life sex with a loved partner can be as good as or better than cybersex, despite its intensity and novelty. But real intimacy takes dedicated work, communication, and play.

Notes

CHAPTER 1: INTRODUCTION TO THE WORLD OF CYBERSEX

1. John Markoff, "A Newer, Lonelier Crowd Emerges in Internet Study," *New York Times*, 16 February 2000, 1.

2. Ibid.

3. Frederick S. Lane III, *Obscene Profits: The Entrepreneurs of Pornography in the Cyber Age* (New York: Routledge, 2000), 123.

4. A. Cooper, D. E. Putnam, L. A. Planchon, and S. C. Boies, "Online Sexual Compulsivity: Getting Tangled in the Net," *Sexual Addiction and Compulsivity* 6 (1999): 79–104. A. Cooper, D. L. Delmonico, and R. Burg, "Cybersex Users, Abusers, and Compulsives: New Findings and Implications," *Sexual Addiction and Compulsivity* 7 (2000): 5–20.

5. Cooper, Putnam, Planchon, and Boies, "Online Sexual Compulsivity," 79–104.

6. Cooper, Delmonico, and Burg, "Cybersex Users, Abusers, and Compulsives," 5–29.

7. Computerworld 1998. Commerce by numbers—Internet population [online]. Available: http://www.computerworld.com/home/Emmerce.nsf/All/pop.

8. Cooper, Delmonico, and Burg, "Cybersex Users, Abusers, and Compulsives," 5–29.

9. Reuters News Service, quoted by Robert McGarvey, rjm@mcgarvey.net, 6 October 1999.

10. *Newsweek*, 31 May 1999, 70.

11. Mark Fritz and Solomon Moore, "Child Porn Raids Lead to Suicides," *Los Angeles Times*, 23 October 1998, A1.

12. *New York Times*, 25 August 1999, A1.

13. Kimberly S. Young, *Caught in the Net: How to Recognize the Signs of Internet Addiction—and a Winning Strategy for Recovery* (New York: John Wiley and Sons, 1998).

CHAPTER 2: WHEN TOO MUCH SEX IS NOT ENOUGH

1. Patrick Carnes, "Understanding Sexual Addiction," *Core Lab Training Manual*, 1992.

2. Patrick Carnes, *Out of the Shadows: Understanding Sexual Addiction* (Minneapolis: CompCare Publications, 1983).

3. G. T. Blanchard, "Differential Diagnosis of Sex Offenders: Distinguishing Characteristics of the Sex Addict," *American Journal of Preventive Psychiatry and Neurology* 2 (1991): 45–47.

4. Richard Irons and Jennifer Schneider, *The Wounded Healer: Addiction-Sensitive Approach to the Sexually Exploitative Professional* (Northvale, N.J.: Jason Aronson Publishers, 1999).

5. A. Cooper, D. L. Delmonico, and R. Burg, "Cybersex Users, Abusers, and Compulsives: New Findings and Implications," *Sexual Addiction and Compulsivity* 7 (2000): 12.

6. Ibid.

CHAPTER 3: CYBERSEX OUT OF CONTROL

1. J. P. Schneider, "Effects of Cybersex Addiction on the Family: Results of a Survey," *Sexual Addiction and Compulsivity* 7 (2000): 31–58.

2. A. Cooper, D. E. Putnam, L. A. Planchon, and S. C. Boies, "Online Sexual Compulsivity: Getting Tangled in the Net," *Sexual Addiction and Compulsivity* 6 (1999): 79–104.

CHAPTER 4: FANTASY AND ROMANCE ADDICTION ON THE INTERNET

1. Meghan Daum, "Virtual Love," *The New Yorker*, 25 August 1997.

2. Robert A. Johnson, *We: Understanding the Psychology of Romantic Love* (San Francisco: Harper San Francisco, 1985), xii.

3. Ellyn Bader and Peter T. Pearson, *In Quest of the Mythical Mate: A Developmental Approach to Diagnosis and Treatment in Couples Therapy* (New York: Brunner/Mazel, 1988).

4. P. Carnes, D. Nonemaker, and N. Skilling, "Gender Differences in Normal and Sexually Addicted Populations," *American Journal of Preventive Psychiatry and Neurology* 3 (1991): 16–23.

5. Ibid.

6. Jennifer Schneider, "A Qualitative Study of Cybersex Participants: Gender Differences, Recovery Issues, and Implications for Therapists." *Sexual Addiction and Compulsivity* (2001, in press).

CHAPTER 5: THE CYBERSEX WIDOW(ER)

1. Jennifer P. Schneider, "Cybersex Addiction: Effect on the Family," *Sexual Addiction and Compulsivity* 7 (2000): 31–58.

2. Jennifer P. Schneider, M. Deborah Corley, and Richard R. Irons, "Surviving Disclosure of Infidelity: Results of an International Survey of 164 Recovering Sex Addicts and Partners," *Sexual Addiction and Compulsivity* 5 (1998): 189–217.

CHAPTER 8: FINDING HELP

1. James O. Prochaska, John C. Norcross, Carlos C. DiClemente, *Changing for Good: A Revolutionary Six-Stage Program for Overcoming Bad Habits and Moving Your Life Positively Forward* (New York: William Morrow and Co., 1994).

Index

◻ ◻ ◻

ABOUT THE AUTHORS

Jennifer P. Schneider, M.D., Ph.D., lives in Tucson, Arizona, where she practices internal medicine and addiction medicine. She received a bachelor's degree in genetics from Cornell University, received a master's degree and a Ph.D. from the University of Michigan in the Department of Human Genetics, and graduated from the University of Arizona College of Medicine. She is certified by the American Board of Internal Medicine and the American Society of Addiction Medicine.

The 1998 recipient of the Patrick Carnes Award for lifetime contribution to advancement of the sex addiction field, Dr. Schneider is the author of two books about the family perspective on sex addiction: *Back from Betrayal: Recovering from His Affairs* (second edition, Recovery Resources Press, 2001) and, with Burt Schneider, *Sex, Lies, and Forgiveness: Couples Speak on Healing from Sex Addiction* (second edition, Recovery Resources Press, 1999). She also wrote *The Wounded Healer: An Addiction-Sensitive Approach to the Sexually Exploitative Professional* (Jason Aronson Publishers, 1999), coauthored with Richard Irons, M.D.

Dr. Schneider serves as the associate editor of *Sexual Addiction and Compulsivity: The Journal of Treatment and Prevention.* She has appeared on numerous television and radio shows. To learn about her other publications, visit her Web site at: **www.jenniferschneider.com.** You can write her at jennifer@jenniferschneider.com.

You can also contact Dr. Schneider at:

Jennifer Schneider, M.D.
Arizona Community Physicians
1500 North Wilmot Road
Tucson, AZ 85712
Tel: (520) 721-7886

Robert Weiss, M.S.W., C.A.S., is currently the clinical director of the Sexual Recovery Institute in Los Angeles. A graduate of the UCLA School of Clinical Social Work, he spent four years as an inpatient sexual addiction specialist training under the direction of Patrick Carnes, Ph.D. Mr. Weiss is an invited clinical educator for the Department of Psychiatry at Harbor-UCLA, the Society for Clinical Social Work, Pepperdine, USC and Antioch Universities, Kaiser Permenente, and numerous clinical and addiction agencies.

Mr. Weiss is a current board member and committee chair of the National Council on Sexual Addiction and Compulsivity. Recently, *ABC World News Tonight*, the *New York Daily News*, the *Washington Post*, and *Newsweek* have interviewed him for his expertise in the area of sexual addiction, and he has served as an addiction consultant to America Online. When not actively seeing patients, he can be found in various places around the United States providing lectures and training on sexual addiction to mental health agencies and corporations. Mr. Weiss can be reached through the Sexual Recovery Institute Web site at **www.sexualrecovery.com.** He resides in southern California.

HAZELDEN INFORMATION AND EDUCATIONAL SERVICES is a division of the Hazelden Foundation, a not-for-profit organization. Since 1949, Hazelden has been a leader in promoting the dignity and treatment of people afflicted with the disease of chemical dependency.

The mission of the foundation is to improve the quality of life for individuals, families, and communities by providing a national continuum of information, education, and recovery services that are widely accessible; to advance the field through research and training; and to improve our quality and effectiveness through continuous improvement and innovation.

Stemming from that, the mission of this division is to provide quality information and support to people wherever they may be in their personal journey—from education and early intervention, through treatment and recovery, to personal and spiritual growth.

Although our treatment programs do not necessarily use everything Hazelden publishes, our bibliotherapeutic materials support our mission and the Twelve Step philosophy upon which it is based. We encourage your comments and feedback.

The headquarters of the Hazelden Foundation are in Center City, Minnesota. Additional treatment facilities are located in Chicago, Illinois; New York, New York; Plymouth, Minnesota; St. Paul, Minnesota; and West Palm Beach, Florida. At these sites, we provide a continuum of care for men and women of all ages. Our Plymouth facility is designed specifically for youth and families.

For more information on Hazelden, please call **1-800-257-7800.** Or you may access our World Wide Web site on the Internet at **http://www.hazelden.org.**